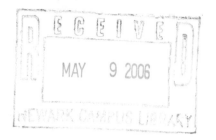

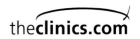

NURSING CLINICS OF NORTH AMERICA

School-Based Health Centers and Nurse-Managed Health Centers

GUEST EDITORS
Judith Scully, PhD, RN, CCNS, and
Diana Hackbarth, PhD, RN, FAAN
and
Barbara Rideout, MSN, APRN, BC

December 2005 • Volume 40 • Number 4

SAUNDERS

An Imprint of Elsevier, Inc.
PHILADELPHIA   LONDON   TORONTO   MONTREAL   SYDNEY   TOKYO

W.B. SAUNDERS COMPANY
A Division of Elsevier Inc.

1600 John F. Kennedy Blvd., Suite 1800, Philadelphia, PA 19103-2899

http://www.theclinics.com

THE NURSING CLINICS OF NORTH AMERICA   Volume 40, Number 4
December 2005   ISSN 0029-6465
Editor: Maria Lorusso   ISBN 1-4160-2739-4

The ideas and opinions expressed in *The Nursing Clinics of North America* do not necessarily reflect those of the Publisher. The Publisher does not assume any responsibility for any injury and/or damage to persons or property arising out of or related to any use of the material contained in this periodical. The reader is advised to check the appropriate medical literature and the product information currently provided by the manufacturer of each drug to be administered to verify the dosage, the method and duration of administration, or contraindications. It is the responsibility of the treating physician or other health care professional, relying on independent experience and knowledge of the patient, to determine drug dosages and the best treatment for the patient. Mention of any product in this issue should not be construed as endorsement by the contributors, editors, or the Publisher of the product or manufacturers' claims.

The Nursing Clinics of North America (ISSN 0029-6465) is published quarterly by Elsevier Inc., Corporate and Editorial Offices: Elsevier Inc., 1600 John F. Kennedy Blvd., Suite 1800, Philadelphia, PA 19103-2899. Accounting and Circulation Offices: 6277 Sea Harbor Drive, Orlando, FL 32887-4800. Periodicals postage paid at Orlando, FL 32862, and additional mailing offices. Subscription price per year is, $105.00 (US individuals), $200.00 (US institutions), $170.00 (international individuals), $240.00 (international institutions), $145.00 (Canadian individuals), $240.00 (Canadian institutions), $55.00 (US students), and $85.00 (international students). To receive student/resident rate, orders must be accompanied by name of affiliated institution, date of term, and the signature of program/residency coordinator on institution letterhead. Orders will be billed at individual rate until proof of status is received. Foreign air speed delivery is included in all *Clinics* subscription prices. All prices are subject to change without notice. POSTMASTER: Send address changes to W.B. Saunders Company, Periodicals Fulfillment, Orlando, FL 32887-4800. **Customer Service: 1-800-654-2452 (US). From outside of the US, call 1-407-345-4000.**

Nursing Clinics of North America is covered in *EMBASE/Excerpta Medica, Index Medicus, Social Sciences Citation Index, Current Contents, ASCA, Cumulative Index to Nursing, RNdex Top 100,* and *Allied Health Literature and International Nursing Index (INI).*

Printed in the United States of America.

ELSEVIER
SAUNDERS

NURSING CLINICS
OF NORTH AMERICA

School-Based Health Centers

GUEST EDITORS

JUDITH SCULLY, PhD, RN, CCNS, Associate Professor, Loyola University Chicago, Niehoff School of Nursing, Chicago, Illinois

DIANA HACKBARTH, PhD, RN, FAAN, Professor, Loyola University Chicago, Niehoff School of Nursing, Chicago, Illinois

CONTRIBUTORS

BRENDA BANNOR, MEd, Partner, Millennia Consulting, Chicago, Illinois

LAURA C. BREY, MS, Associate Director, National Assembly on School-Based Health Care, Raleigh, North Carolina

TERESA K. DAVIS, APN, MSN, WHNP, Clinical Nurse Manager, Loyola University Chicago, Niehoff School of Nursing, Chicago, Illinois

BETH EDWARDS, RN, MSN, BC, FNP, Clinical Nurse Manager, Health Care Centers in Schools/Coordinated School Health Services, Baton Rouge, Louisiana

GAIL B. GALL, RN, MSN, Loyola University Chicago, Niehoff School of Nursing, Chicago, Illinois

LINDA GILLILAND, PhD, ARNP, CPNP, Total Family Health Care, Clermont, Florida

ELAINE M. GUSTAFSON, MSN, RN, CS, PNP, Assistant Professor, Yale University School of Nursing, New Haven, Connecticut

DIANA HACKBARTH, PhD, RN, FAAN, Professor, Loyola University Chicago, Niehoff School of Nursing, Chicago, Illinois

CAROLYN R. MONTFORD, PsyD, Assistant Professor, Department of Psychiatry, Division of Psychology, Stritch School of Medicine, Loyola University Medical Center, Chicago, Illinois

SUSAN M. MURRAY, RN, MPH, Program Coordinator, School Health Programs, Swedish Covenant Hospital, Chicago, Illinois

HENRY J. PERKINS, PhD, Northwestern University, Counseling and Psychological Services, Evanston, Illinois

CAROLYN READ, MPH, MSW, Health Educator, Loyola University Chicago, Niehoff School of Nursing, Chicago, Illinois

JUDITH SCULLY, PhD, RN, CCNS, Associate Professor, Loyola University Chicago, Niehoff School of Nursing, Chicago, Illinois

DEIDRE M. WASHINGTON, MPH, CHES, Program Manager, National Assembly on School-Based Health Care, Washington, District of Columbia

VALERIE WEBB, MPH, Assistant Health Officer, Cook County Department of Public Health, Oak Park, Illinois

ELSEVIER
SAUNDERS

NURSING CLINICS
OF NORTH AMERICA

Nurse-Managed Health Centers

GUEST EDITOR

BARBARA RIDEOUT, MSN, APRN, BC, Assistant Professor and Track Coordinator, Family Nurse Practitioner Program, Drexel University College of Nursing and Health Professions, Philadelphia, Pennsylvania

CONTRIBUTORS

LAURA ANDERKO, RN, PhD, Associate Dean for Practice and Associate Professor, College of Nursing, University of Wisconsin-Milwaukee, Milwaukee, Wisconsin

CLAUDIA BARTZ, RN, PhD, FAAN, Associate Clinical Professor, College of Nursing, University of Wisconsin-Milwaukee, Milwaukee, Wisconsin

RITA BEAM, RN, MSN, Director of Professional Development, National Nurse Family Partnership, Denver, Colorado

SUSAN M. BEIDLER, PhD, MBE, ARNP, BC, Research Assistant Professor, Quantum Foundation Center for Innovation in School and Community Well Being, Christine E. Lynn College of Nursing, Florida Atlantic University, Boca Raton, Florida

SUSAN BRAUN, MS, APRN, BC, Director, Center for Integrated Health Care, University of Illinois at Chicago College of Nursing, Department of Public Health, Mental Health, and Administrative Nursing, Chicago, Illinois

LINDA CAMPBELL, PhD, RN, Assistant Professor and Chair of Curriculum Committee, Loretto Heights Department of Nursing, Rueckert-Hartman School for Health Professions, Regis University, Denver, Colorado

MICHELLE CARR, RN, BSN, Community Health Nurse, University of North Carolina Nursing Center for Health Promotion, Charlotte, North Carolina

KATY DAWLEY, PhD, CNM, Assistant Professor, Drexel University College of Nursing and Health Professions, Philadelphia, Pennsylvania

ANNE FERRARI, PhD, RN, Associate Professor, Drexel University College of Nursing and Health Professions, Philadelphia, Pennsylvania

BETHANY HALL-LONG, PhD, RNC, FAAN, Associate Professor, School of Nursing, College of Health Sciences, University of Delaware, Newark, Delaware

TINE HANSEN-TURTON, MGA, Executive Director, National Nursing Centers Consortium, Philadelphia, Pennsylvania

EVELYN R. HAYES, PhD, APRN, BC, Professor, School of Nursing, College of Health Sciences, University of Delaware, Newark, Delaware

SALLY LUNDEEN, RN, PhD, FAAN, Dean and Professor, College of Nursing, University of Wisconsin-Milwaukee, Milwaukee, Wisconsin

LUCY MARION, PhD, RN, FAAN, Dean and Professor, School of Nursing, Medical College of Georgia, Augusta, Georgia

JUDITH McDEVITT, PhD, APRN, BC, Clinical Assistant Professor, University of Illinois at Chicago College of Nursing, Department of Public Health, Mental Health, and Administrative Nursing, Chicago, Illinois

MARGARET NOYES, ND, APRN, BC, Clinical Instructor, University of Illinois at Chicago College of Nursing, Department of Public Health, Mental Health, and Administrative Nursing, Chicago, Illinois

LISA ANN PLOWFIELD, RN, PhD, Professor and Chair, School of Nursing, College of Health Sciences, University of Delaware, Newark, Delaware

BARBARA RIDEOUT, MSN, APRN, BC, Assistant Professor and Track Coordinator, Family Nurse Practitioner Program, Drexel University College of Nursing and Health Professions, Philadelphia, Pennsylvania

MARSHA SNYDER, PhD, APRN, BC, Clinical Assistant Professor, University of Illinois at Chicago College of Nursing, Department of Public Health, Mental Health, and Administrative Nursing, Chicago, Illinois

YVONNE YOUSEY, RN, CPNP, PhD, Assistant Professor, Department of Family and Community Nursing, University of North Carolina at Charlotte, Charlotte, North Carolina

NURSING CLINICS
OF NORTH AMERICA

School-Based Health Centers

> SBHCs are filling a gap in health care needs for many of our nation's children. They provide services to an underserved population of children and adolescents, focusing on provision of health services and the promotion of health through population-based education programs. Schools with SBHCs are finding that significant physical, mental, and dental health issues are being addressed during the school day, allowing children to remain in school. The mission of SBHCs to contribute to the health of children by providing access to primary health care and preventive health care services is being actualized.

> School-based health centers (SBHCs) are a growing phenomenon in the United States and appear to be an ideal fit for school of nursing (SON) sponsorship. However, nationally only about 6% of existing SBHCs are sponsored by either an SON or a school of medicine. Sponsorship of health care in schools is consistent with the mission of university-based SONs, but also presents many challenges. Despite these challenges, the authors believe that the benefit to nursing students, faculty, and the profession far outweigh constraints. This article describes the many benefits that can occur when SONs create and maintain a SBHC in their own community. Extensive practical suggestions for how to overcome the barriers that constrain university faculty from developing service-oriented programs in the community are also emphasized.

> To facilitate the successful implementation of school-based health centers (SBHCs), funding streams and technical assistance are needed from various resources. The core funding models for service delivery

include federal grants, state grants, local funding, community partnerships, foundations, and patient revenue. Technical assistance opportunities are available through professional organizations, SBHC associations, state health departments, and primary care associations at the national and state levels. This article explores the various federal, state, and local funding sources, and the technical assistance resources and opportunities available to SBHCs and their staff.

School-based health centers provide accessible quality health services to culturally diverse student populations. Numerous challenges exist in providing culturally competent services in a school setting. This article presents models of culturally competent care, practice recommendations, and practical resources in an attempt to improve the provision of culturally competent services. In addition, one school health center's initiative to outreach culturally diverse students into health careers is highlighted.

School-based health centers in high schools provide a unique setting in which to deliver risk-reduction and resilience-building services to adolescents. The traditional health care system operating in the United States focuses on the treatment of illness and disease rather than on preventing problems originating from health risk behaviors. Nurse practitioners can promote healthy behavior in adolescents through linkages to parents, schools, and community organizations; by conducting individual risk assessments; and by providing health education and access to creative health programs that build resilience and promote protective factors. With a focus on wellness, nurse practitioners as advanced practice nurses and specialists in disease prevention and health promotion can establish students' health priorities in the context of the primary health care they deliver on a daily basis.

Although the incidence of childhood obesity is rising at an alarming rate, weight loss programs for children are few and often inaccessible for various reasons, including cost, transportation difficulties, and lack of parental involvement. School-based programs, offered free of charge, make weight management more accessible. School-based health centers have a unique opportunity to assure that schools stay in the forefront of obesity prevention and management. This article discusses one such program that was designed and implemented by the staff of a Louisiana school-based health center.

School-based health centers (SBHCs) emerged in the late 1960s as a response to concerns about the health care needs of undeserved children and adolescents who were often left out of the health care system. Most SBHCs provide an array of primary health care services such as routine health screenings, immunizations, acute care for common conditions, behavioral risk assessments, and health education on various topics. One of the most important functions of an SBHC is the provision of psychological services for teenagers experiencing depression, adjustment difficulties, substance abuse, and trauma. SBHCs may also serve as an important resource for those students affected by violence through the provision of crisis intervention, grief counseling, and on-going violence prevention education.

Prevention programs are a valuable component of the comprehensive services offered at school-based health centers (SBHC). Reducing risky adolescent behaviors is an effective way to reduce the morbidity and mortality burden among the school-age population. Programs using peer educators and youth-initiated websites can increase knowledge and self-esteem and help reduce risky sexual behaviors. Because many SBHCs provide services beyond traditional primary care, there is great need to support and increase the number of SBHC prevention programs targeted at communities at risk.

Problems that affect the health and well-being of the nation's children and youth are becoming increasingly complex and interrelated, requiring the joint efforts of education, health, and social service systems. School-based health centers (SBHCs) provide a bridge between these disciplines. Professionals who staff SBHCs routinely interface with key partners within their host schools. This article provides lessons from the field, exploring the intricacies of the collaborative process from the perspective of 17 nurse practitioners working in an SBHC in Cook County, Illinois.

The goal of school-based health centers (SBHCs) is to provide culturally competent primary, preventive, and mental health care services for students who otherwise may not have access to care. Often, an SBHC is the primary health care provider for students because many adolescents are uninsured or lack access to other health care service providers. At other times, the SBHC works in collaboration with primary care providers and other health professionals to provide health care services for students and their families. Complex health and social problems and changes in professional practice make it impossible to serve clients effectively without collaborating with professionals from other disciplines. One process used in SBHCs to assure that students' needs and concerns are addressed is an interdisciplinary case review (ICR). The ICR is a method of evaluating complex cases with members of the health care team to ensure that the physical and mental health and social needs of students are meeting or exceeding the standard of care.

Evaluation and dissemination of the outcomes of school-based health center (SBHC) services is essential for the continual growth and funding of SBHCs in the United States. Since their inception, SBHCs have been practice sites for nurse practitioners and have used interdisciplinary teams to provide care for underserved school-aged children. Early research and evaluation focused on describing the types of services and the quality of care provided. Supporters of SBHCs were anxious to demonstrate that the care provided was "as good as" care delivered in traditional primary care practices. Documentation of program impacts, such as changes in population health indicators or improved academic achievement, has been more elusive. Current evaluation priorities outlined by the National Assembly on School-Based Health Care include evaluation of mental health services using a new online tool; assessing productivity of SBHC staff; measuring quality; and attempts to link SBHC care with improved academic outcomes.

NURSING CLINICS
OF NORTH AMERICA

Nurse-Managed Health Centers

Nurse-managed health centers are critical safety net providers. Increasing support of these centers is a promising strategy for the federal government to reduce health disparities. To continue as safety net providers, nurse-managed health centers need to receive equal compensation as other federally funded providers. Ultimately, the long-term sustainability of nurse-managed centers rests on prospective payments or similar federally mandated funding mechanisms.

Community-based nurse-managed practice (CBNMP) brings primary health care to local, typically vulnerable, populations. Despite cost-effective, high quality care, a 21% decline in academic CBNMPs was documented in the 1990s. A multiple case study addressed factors that hindered or facilitated diffusion and sustainability of CBNMPs in prevalent practice settings. To promote sustainable practice, CBNMPs should articulate a practice mission, identify the practice as nursing, create a team approach, balance mission with margin, and promote attractive sites. Other recommendations include planning for growth and evolution of health care and applying for awards to increase the visibility and political clout of CBNMPs.

Practice-based research networks (PBRNs) can provide a range of opportunities for nurses working in primary care settings. This article reports on the early experiences of the Midwest Nursing Centers Consortium Research Network (MNCCRN), one of only two nursing PBRNs in the nation. Findings from the MNCCRN's first research study, Wellness for a Lifetime, indicate success with implementing research across geographically distant sites, and positive client outcomes related to improving nutrition and physical activity. Lessons learned in establishing a PBRN and implementing research studies in the real world are described as well as challenges for the future.

Ethical issues are commonplace in the health care delivery system. Nurse practitioners (NPs) working in nurse-managed health centers (NMHCs) frequently care for patients who are vulnerable and marginalized as a result of their culture, language, low income, or lack of insurance. Because a nurse's commitment is to care for patients without considerations of social or economic status, personal attributes, or the nature of health problems, the distress that occurs while advocating for patients through and around existing barriers to health care access needs to be anticipated and addressed.

Historically, public health nurses have been the cornerstone of keeping communities healthy. Ideally, primary care is the point of access for health care and nurse practitioners provide cost-effective, high quality primary care. It is a natural progression to build a nurse-managed health center on the foundation of public health nursing with primary care provided by nurse practitioners. Such collaboration produced the 11th Street Family Health Services of Drexel University serving the most vulnerable census tracts in Pennsylvania.

Nurse-managed centers have been at the forefront of providing ambulatory care alternatives for underserved populations lacking access to care. Following this model, the Center for Integrated Health Care of the College of Nursing at the University of Illinois in Chicago delivers primary and mental health care services to a population of people with serious and persistent mental illness. The authors' experience illustrates the many rewards and challenges that nurse-managed centers face. This article describes their center's model of integrated care, examines selected performance indicators, and discusses the implications, opportunities, and challenges ahead.

NURSING CLINICS
OF NORTH AMERICA

THE CLINICS ARE NOW AVAILABLE ONLINE!

Access your subscription at:
http://www.theclinics.com

Nurs Clin N Am 40 (2005) xv–xvii

NURSING CLINICS
OF NORTH AMERICA

ELSEVIER
SAUNDERS

PREFACE

School-Based Health Centers

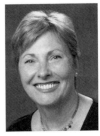 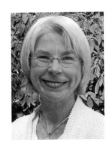

Judith Scully, PhD, RN, CCNS, Diana Hackbarth, PhD, RN, FAAN
Guest Editors

Over 30 years ago, poor access to health care, troubling statistics on risky health behaviors, and unintended pregnancy among teens motivated health care professionals, community health care leaders, and school administrators to create the first primary health care programs in schools—school-based health centers [1]. Today, there are approximately 1500 school-based health centers across the United States providing on-site primary health care, mental health, and preventive health services to help students stay healthy and maximize their opportunities to learn [2].

This issue of the *Nursing Clinics of North America* focuses on the unique contributions of school-based health centers. Our intent is to introduce and reintroduce readers to a model of comprehensive health care delivered in a setting most familiar and accessible to children and young people—their schools. School-based health centers provide access to health care for children and youth who lack or have insufficient health insurance. School-based health centers also address unmet health needs. It is estimated that 12.5% of children and youth between the ages of 5 and 17 years have unmet health needs as compared with 6% of children 0 to 4 years with unmet medical needs [3].

The initial section of this issue lays the foundation of school-based health centers. The past is presented; the present is outlined, including the types of services, sponsorships, and funding sources available for school-based health centers; and the future is discussed. Opportunities and challenges for schools of nursing, academic health centers, hospitals, and health departments who may wish to develop new school-based health centers are addressed.

0029-6465/05/$ – see front matter
doi:10.1016/j.cnur.2005.08.012

Federal, state, private foundation, patient revenue, and community partnerships are potential funding streams that could facilitate the successful implementation of a school-based health center. Readers are provided with an overview of the technical assistance available to new sponsors of school-based health centers, funding opportunities available to sustain existing school-based health centers, and a variety of evaluation strategies to measure quality of care and outcomes for school-based health centers.

Nursing has a long history of providing care to children and adolescents in school settings. Changes in the philosophy of school health services, the role of school nurses, and the role of emergent advanced practice nursing supported the development and expansion of school-based health centers. The second section of this issue provides articles on the distinctions between the roles of advanced practice nurses and school nurses as well as the partnerships that exist between education and health care. School-based health centers are unique for many reasons. The school-age population reflects the growing diversity in the United States. School-based health centers provide nursing students, nurse practitioner students, medical students, psychology students, and dietetic students an arena in which to practice culturally sensitive, interdisciplinary health care and to appreciate the strengths, qualities, and talents of students from culturally diverse backgrounds. Another important element of school-based health care is the close link to the larger community. Continuity of care, use of community resources, and parental involvement are hallmarks of school-based health care.

The large majority of school-based health centers are located in lower-income areas in both urban and rural settings. The problems associated with poverty—physical, mental, emotional, familial, and societal problems—are obstacles to school success for many children and adolescents [4]. Several topics in this issue mirror the concerns and challenges of society to emergent societal problems such as violence, obesity, and sexually transmitted infections such as HIV/AIDS. School-based health centers are often venues for model programs that address health risk behaviors that adversely impact children and adolescents' health. In a school-based health center, health promotion and disease prevention activities are stressed, as are asset-confirming models that promote resiliency and help students to develop positive self-worth and reach their full potential. Health professionals in school-based health centers are knowledgeable and "user friendly" in meeting student needs. Interactions with providers are designed to empower students to develop the skills, awareness, and knowledge necessary to become experts on their own health.

Today, nurses and other health professionals have an opportunity to promote the health of children and youth and engage in strategies to develop healthy, positive, lifelong behaviors. School-based health centers provide creative alternatives to the traditional health care delivery model. They improve the physical and emotional health of students, promote healthy lifestyles, and provide available, accessible primary care and preventive health care year 12 months a year. We are proud to present this series of articles that highlight the various aspects of school-based health centers throughout the United States and thank the authors for their diligence and thoughtfulness in researching and writing the articles that appear in this issue of the *Nursing Clinics of North America*.

Judith Scully, PhD, RN, CCNS
Diana Hackbarth, PhD, RN, FAAN
Niehoff School of Nursing
Loyola University Chicago
6525 North Sheridan Road
Chicago, IL 60611, USA

E-mail addresses: jscully@wpo.it.luc.edu (J. Scully);
dhackba@luc.edu (D. Hackbarth)

References

[1] National Assembly on School Based Health Care. Creating access to care for children and youth: school based health center census 1998–1999. Washington, DC: National Assembly on School Based Health Care; June 2000.

[2] National Assembly on School Based Health Care. Available at: www.nasbhc.org. Accessed June 17, 2005.

[3] US Department of Health and Human Services, Health Resources Service Administration. Improving Health of Mothers and Children. Washington, DC: US Department of Health and Human Services; 1998.

[4] Cotton K. School-Community collaboration: improving life for urban youth and their families. Prevention First: Prevention Forum 1997;17:6–11.

Nurs Clin N Am 40 (2005) 595–606

NURSING CLINICS
OF NORTH AMERICA

ELSEVIER
SAUNDERS

History and Overview of School-Based Health Centers in the US

Elaine M. Gustafson, MSN, RN, CS, PNP

Yale University School of Nursing, 100 Church Street South, P.O. Box 9740, New Haven, CT 06536, USA

According to the World Health Organization (WHO), primary health care is the cornerstone of health care delivery and many countries are seeking creative ways to adapt primary care services to health and social issues. WHO further argues that the goals of health systems include increasing not only the level of health of the population but also the level of responsiveness of the health system to the legitimate expectations and needs of people [1]. Thus, it can be said that school-based health centers (SBHCs) are an idea whose time has come. They provide services to an underserved population of children and adolescents, focusing on provision of health services and the promotion of health through population-based education programs.

"The mission of a School-Based Health Center is to provide comprehensive health education, as well as primary medical, reproductive and mental health services to enrolled students" [2]. SBHCs offer preventive, innovative initiatives and provide access to health care for many youth. SBHCs have significantly increased in number in the past 12 years in the United States (Fig. 1). In 1990, there were 200 centers located in 45 states plus the District of Columbia. In 2002, there were over 1500 school-based, school-linked, and mobile school health centers [3]. According to the most recent state statistics compiled in 2002 by the National Assembly for School-Based Health Care (NASBHC), SBHCs are found in urban (61%), rural (27%), and suburban (12%) areas and are predominantly nurse managed with nurse practitioners or physicians working full-time in 54% of health centers and part-time (25 hours or less per week) in the remaining health centers [3].

SBHCs are staffed by a multidisciplinary team of nurse practitioners or physician's assistants, physicians, mental health providers, and other support staff. This support staff may include nurses, health educators, outreach workers, medical assistants, substance abuse counselors, dental hygienists, nutritionists, and others.

E-mail address: elaine.gustafson@yale.edu

0029-6465/05/$ – see front matter
doi:10.1016/j.cnur.2005.08.001

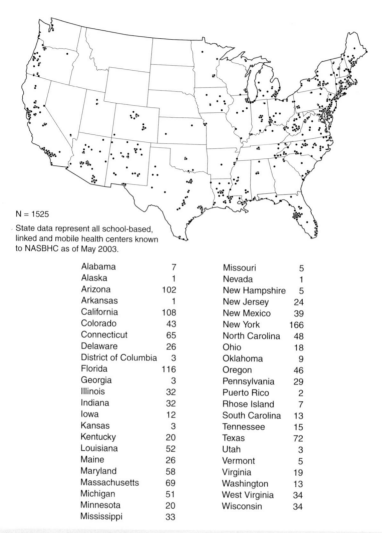

N = 1525

State data represent all school-based,
linked and mobile health centers known
to NASBHC as of May 2003.

Alabama	7	Missouri	5
Alaska	1	Nevada	1
Arizona	102	New Hampshire	5
Arkansas	1	New Jersey	24
California	108	New Mexico	39
Colorado	43	New York	166
Connecticut	65	North Carolina	48
Delaware	26	Ohio	18
District of Columbia	3	Oklahoma	9
Florida	116	Oregon	46
Georgia	3	Pennsylvania	29
Illinois	32	Puerto Rico	2
Indiana	32	Rhose Island	7
Iowa	12	South Carolina	13
Kansas	3	Tennessee	15
Kentucky	20	Texas	72
Louisiana	52	Utah	3
Maine	26	Vermont	5
Maryland	58	Virginia	19
Massachusetts	69	Washington	13
Michigan	51	West Virginia	34
Minnesota	20	Wisconsin	34
Mississippi	33		

Fig. 1. SBHCs in the United States.

Appendices 1 through 3 depict some common problems of illness, family disruption, and emotional distress experienced by children enrolled in SBHCs. Children who are ill or suffering emotional trauma cannot learn to their full potential. The three vignettes are examples of ways a SBHC links health and education by providing accessible primary health care and mental health services to children and adolescents in need.

ORIGINS OF SCHOOL-BASED HEALTH CENTERS

The American Academy of Pediatrics, through its Community Access to Child Health (CATCH) program, fostered the development of the first SBHCs. These opened in the late 1960s and early 1970s and were organized by a local pediatrician, Philip J. Porter, MD. One of the earliest health centers was in an elementary school in Cambridge, Mass. Four other health centers also opened in that city followed by health centers in Dallas and Minneapolis-St. Paul. These early initiatives formed the foundation for SBHCs in the United States [4].

In 1978, funding through the Robert Wood Johnson Foundation (RWJF) provided the impetus to increase the numbers SBHCs throughout the United States [5]. This initiative spurred local efforts by policy makers at the state level to fund SBHCs. In Connecticut, Governor Lowell Weicker called for a SBHC in every school and when he left office in 1995 nearly 50 clinics were established [6]. In 1995, the Health Resource & Service Administration initiated a program to provide grant funding for SBHCs. More recently, Senator Joseph Lieberman proposed the expansion of the national network of SBHCs to increase preventive health care services to children [7].

In contrast to this rather recent innovation of the provision of primary health care services in schools, the history of school nursing in the United States dates back more than 100 years. The first school nurse, Lina Rogers, was employed in New York City in 1902 by Lillian Wald of the Henry Street Settlement (Table 1). Her role was to address the large number of children excluded from school for communicable diseases and to educate parents, teachers, and children about disease control and prevention. She also made home visits to follow up on children to facilitate early recovery and return to school. Administrators were so impressed with the decline in the number of absent students that they began to hire school nurses [8].

Over the next few decades, the role of the school nurse broadened to include health education in addition to medical inspection and examination. According to Wold [8], this broadening of roles for the school nurse led to an overextension of services and role confusion with mixed allegiances to public health and education. By the 1950s, health education was the major responsibility of school nurses. School nurses provided one-on-one counseling with students and parents, in-service education for classroom teachers, and leadership in developing family life education. School health services that were offered consisted primarily of meeting state mandates concerning immunization and screenings. Early identification of health problems was designed to improve child health through case finding and referral to community physicians [8].

By the 1960s, social change was in the air with a proliferation of welfare and health programs. Recognition of the needs of the handicapped child in regular education came to the forefront. In 1974, The Education for All Handicapped Children Act was passed. This landmark legislation led to the mainstreaming of handicapped children into regular classrooms and broadened the role of the school nurse. The expertise of nurses was needed to advocate for special needs children. Nurses suddenly were responsible for children who had physical and developmental disabilities and severe chronic health problems previously not known in the school setting.

Table 1
Evolution of school nursing/SBHCs

	1900–1905	1906–1920	1920–1940	1941–1950	1950–1964	1965–1990	1990–present
Political/cultural climate	Massive immigration; women's rights/suffrage	WWI; industrial wealth leads to philanthrophy		WWII	Great Society era 1974: Education for All Handicapped Children Act	ERA	SCHIP
Population health issues	Communicable disease leading cause of death; average life expectancy 47 years		Poor health of recruits; expansion of dental care	Women in the workforce		Increased awareness of mental health concerns	Uninsured and underinsured children
Health care in schools	Lillian Wald founded PH Nursing; first school nurse: Lina Rogers, 1902; school nurse and physician work collaboratively in schools to provide cost-effective treatment (goal: keep kids in school)	School nurse role: medical inspection and examination; Forsythe family establishes dental clinic for children in Boston	SN role broadened to include health education	SN role focus: immunizations; screenings; case finding; referral to community physicians	School Nurse Practitioner Program, Denver, CO	First SBHCs established; proliferation of SBHCs; RWJ funding	Medicaid billing for SHBC; 1995 established NASBHC; NASN 2002 recommended SN ratio 1:750

Abbreviations: ERA, Equal Rights Amendment; NASBHC, National Assembly for School-based Health Care; NASN, National Association for School Nurses; PH, Public Health; RWJF, Robert Wood Johnson Foundation; SCHIP, State Children's Health Insurance Plan; SN, School Nurse; WW, World War.

Despite the growing need for more expert health professionals in schools, school nurses faced budget cuts, challenging their once-secure position and leading to loss of job security [9]. The number of school nursing positions nationwide continued to decrease. Loretta Ford attributed this decrease to the failure of nurses to vocalize the worth of nursing services to school boards, administrators, and consumers [10].

At the end of the 1970s, proposals to expand the scope and efficiency of school health services were emerging. There was continued dissatisfaction with the limited role of the school nurse and school health services. Igoe [11] reports that the public was no longer content with simply the identification of health problems at school. Instead they wanted diagnosis and treatment as part of a school health program. To meet these public concerns, the School Nurse Practitioner program was established in the mid-1970s in Denver, Colo [11]. This program enabled nurses to become skilled in physical examination, diagnosis, and treatment; areas previously restricted to the role of physicians. The program formed the backdrop for the delivery of primary care in schools, using the advanced practice nurse in conjunction with the school nurse.

SBHCs, although not equivalent to a school health program, have become a rallying point for those who have been dissatisfied with the practice limitations of traditional school health services. Supporters of this vision are primarily health care providers, including school nurses and other health professionals, who worry about the inadequacy of community-based services for adolescents in particular and for poor children of all ages [9]. Early efforts to establish SBHCs met with controversy focusing on issues of reproductive health care and parental rights. Despite these controversies, by the 1990s SBHCs began to grow rapidly [12]. Today in many schools that have SBHCs, the concept of providing health care in the same building in which children attend class is as accepted as having a school library.

Three categories of SBHCs, listed in Box 1, are described in the 2001–2002 survey of SBHCs by the NASBHC [3].

Why school-based health centers?

Access! Access! Access! By 2010, it is estimated that the population of school-aged children (ages 6–17) will reach 48 million [13]. According to the Children's Defense Fund, one in six American children, approximately 8.6 million children, lived below the poverty line in 2003 [14]. Families living in poverty may be single-parent families or families where both parents are employed because of increasing financial pressures, making trips to a health care provider often difficult and sometimes impossible for parents.

Many children are uninsured or underinsured. Although there has been a significant decrease in the number of children under age 18 who do not have health insurance, 9.4% of children (6.9 million) remained uninsured in 2003. Twenty-eight percent of poor and near-poor children rely on public coverage. Hispanic families are the most likely to be uninsured. Uninsured children are

> **Box 1: Three categories of school-based health centers according to the 2001–2002 National Assembly for School-Based Health Care survey**
>
> Primary care model
>
> Clinical services: nurse practitioner or physician's assistant (PA)
>
> Clinical support/education: registered nurse (RN) or licensed practical nurse (LPN)
>
> Optional: social services/dental care
>
> Primary care/mental health combination
>
> Clinical services: NP or PA
>
> Clinical support/education: RN or LPN
>
> Mental health support services: licensed clinical social worker (LCSW) or psychologist/substance abuse counselor
>
> Primary care and mental health plus
>
> Clinical services: NP or PA
>
> Clinical support: RN or LPN
>
> Mental health services: LCSW or psychologist/substance abuse counselor
>
> Social service case workers/nutritionists/dental care

13 times as likely to not have a usual source of health care as children who have private health insurance (27% versus 2%) [15].

Adolescents are the least likely group to seek care at a health provider's office. Because of time constraints and a narrow medical focus, even when adolescents have access to a health care provider, there is often minimal impact on adverse health behavior. Health providers often do not include mental health and health education support, which are important issues for adolescents [16]. Risky health behaviors, including violence, unprotected sex, and substance abuse, contribute to the leading causes of morbidity and mortality for many adolescents [17]. These risky behaviors are often not discussed with traditional health care providers. On the other hand, SBHC providers see risk assessment and addressing unhealthy lifestyle behaviors as a priority in their visits.

SBHCs provide a safety net for parents and children. Teachers and administrators are pleased that SBHC services are available so that issues can be addressed in a timely fashion and students can return to class ready to learn. Active outreach, health promotion, and continuity of care are hallmarks of SHBC care. Children are encouraged to share their anxieties and fears, which may underlie their health concerns. Confidential care is an essential component of health care for teens, and SBHCs remain committed to this principle of care. Parental permission is a requirement for student use of SBHCs, and parental involvement remains a constant goal. SBHCs are an effective way to provide care for underserved children and teens [6]. In addition, SBHCs are unique in that no one is denied care based on their ability to pay.

Types of health services in school-based health centers

According to the NASBHC 2001–2002 Survey of School-Based Health Centers, most SBHCs provide the basics of primary health care. These fundamentals includes health assessments; anticipatory guidance; screenings for vision and hearing; immunizations; acute illness care; and treatment and laboratory services. Of the 1067 health centers surveyed at that time, more than 90% offered acute illness care, including asthma treatment and prescriptions, and screenings for vision, hearing, and scoliosis. More than 80% of health centers provided medications and treatment for chronic illnesses and offered laboratory testing. Dental care was available in 46% of centers with 12% offering dental sealant programs. Although reproductive health services are available in some centers serving middle and high school students, more than three quarters do not dispense contraception on site. Most of these health centers, however, do provide pregnancy testing, family planning counseling, treatment for sexually transmitted diseases, and HIV/AIDS counseling [3]. Those that do not provide reproductive services on site have a referral system in place to refer students to community agencies for these services.

Various on-site mental health services are available to students. Eighty percent of SBHCs provide services that may include individual and group counseling, family therapy consultation, and case management. The most frequent mental health services provided in SBHCs include screening, assessment, referrals, and crisis intervention [3]. Common mental health diagnoses in two large urban SBHCs in operation for over 20 years included posttraumatic stress disorder, anxiety disorder, dysthymia, and adolescent adjustment disorder [18]. In addition, many health centers provide in-service counseling for faculty on issues such as reporting abuse, detecting depression, and maintaining confidentiality.

Prevention and early intervention are key initiatives in SBHCs. Health care providers routinely use screening tools to assess the level of risk for adverse health behaviors, and educate students regarding threats to their health. They also facilitate the development of appropriate skills to avoid high-risk behaviors. Simply taking the time to ask questions about students' health or certain high-risk behaviors may provide the student with the opportunity to talk about problems that might otherwise remain unaddressed. Ultimately, the goal is for students to become educated consumers of health care and to learn to make informed decisions about their health.

A SBHC provides the student with an interdisciplinary team approach through which their issues can be addressed. A student who has asthma may be assessed by the health care provider, treated on-site, and given a prescription for long-term treatment. In addition, a student may be referred to a social worker for assessment of emotional issues related to the asthma. An outreach worker may be available to make a home visit to assist the parent in the removal of asthma triggers in the home. Comprehensive services with regular follow-up is a hallmark of school-based health care. The array of services and close working relationships with the students often prevent students from "falling through the cracks" of the health care system. Community partners are often used for referral and consultation, adding to the comprehensive nature of services.

Health promotion

Health promotion and educational interventions reach well beyond the SBHC into the classroom, school, and community. Prevention and early intervention activities may focus on nutrition and physical activity counseling; tobacco prevention/cessation programs; injury prevention; pregnancy and sexually transmitted infection prevention; and many others. Mental health outreach programs may include interventions to deal with loss and bereavement, bullying prevention, anger management, and violence prevention. Wellness-focused programs may include stress management, meditation, healthy nutrition, and physical activity. Health promotion activities may be held after school, in the evening, or on weekends in the school or the community, or during school hours.

Models of school-based health center sponsorship

According to Julia Lear (personal communication, 2005), Director of the Center for Health and Health Care in Schools, a key factor in differentiating SBHCs from traditional school nursing services is their sponsorship. Most SBHCs function independently of the school in which they are located because they are sponsored by agencies outside of the school. This sponsorship often provides health centers with a strong management structure tied into the sponsoring agencies. For example, the multisite centers (eg, Denver Health in Colorado and Montefiore Hospital in New York City) are especially strong as a result of their ability to spread management costs over a broad base. They maintain strong political support because they serve a large number of children, which provides some assurance of continued state support and thus long-term viability. According to Dr. Lear (personal communication, 2005), "a single School-Based Health Center [is] a 'cut flower,' beautiful in its own right, but what we need are many centers with a strong base like a large plant or tree, well rooted, visible and able to maintain themselves".

Sponsoring agencies are critical to the viability of the centers. Approximately 90% of SBHCs are sponsored by agencies outside of the school district. The NASBHC 2001–2002 survey revealed that the two largest sponsoring agencies are hospital/medical centers and health departments (51%). These are followed by community health centers (18%), nonprofit health organizations (11%), school systems (9%), medical and nursing schools (6%), and others (4%) (Fig. 2). Sponsoring agencies provide human and financial resources to maintain SBHCs. Sponsoring agencies also play a large part in arranging additional funding, helping to secure political support, and aiding in negotiations with the school system.

Most SBHCs are affiliated with large hospitals or comprehensive health centers [3]. These hospitals and health centers may derive many benefits from sponsoring SBHCs. These benefits include gaining a portal into the community, which allows hospital-based trainees (eg, nursing, medical and dental

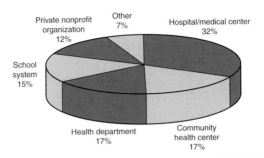

Fig. 2. SBHC sponsoring agencies.

students, mental health providers) to practice in a nontraditional site and experience interdisciplinary practice. Schools of nursing may derive similar benefits from sponsorship of SBHCs. SBHCs can be a venue for advanced practice nursing students to care for children and teens in a nontraditional site, can offer opportunities for interdisciplinary collaboration, and can be a place to actualize nursing models of care. Many health departments sponsor SBHCs, which is consistent with population-based disease prevention mandates of health departments in the United States.

Funding for school-based health centers

Funding for SBHCs comes from various sources, which creates challenges for the sponsoring agencies. There are many advocates for school-based care but they do not speak in concert, leaving SBHCs "somewhat of a political orphan" [19]. The mission of SBHCs may vary from state to state, from providing a medical home for uninsured children to placing emphasis on increasing high school graduation rates. On the state level, grassroots advocacy has played a significant role in some states, leading to strong gubernatorial support and funding through grants and Medicaid managed care revenues [20]. As of June, 1999, 36 states provided SBHC grant support, 43 allowed Medicaid billing, and 22 allowed centers to be providers in Medicaid managed care networks. These developments in financial support mark the transition of SBHCs "from the margins to the mainstream" of the American health care system [19]. However, variability between states makes advocacy for funding on the federal level difficult.

The future of school-based health centers

Currently, only a small percentage of the approximately 90,000 schools in the United States have a SBHC, which presents enormous opportunities and challenges. According to Lear (personal communication, March 4, 2005), the good news is that federal funds for safety net services appear to be expanding with the huge influx of funds for community health centers. Because of this infusion of funds into the community, the number of SBHCs may also increase.

To guarantee the viability of SBHCs, it is critical for the centers to build bridges with potential community partners. Challenges in the new millennium will likely include care of children who have special health care needs; mental health assessment and treatment; poverty; lack of health insurance; and providing medical homes for many children. Evidence-based practice and electronic medical records will be vehicles to increase connections between school health services and the larger health care system.

The positive impact of SBHCs has led to their endorsement by several professional organizations, including the American Nurses Association, the National Association of Pediatric Nurse Practitioners, the National Association of School Nurses, and the National Association of State Nurse Consultants [21]. Other organizations that support SBHCs are the American Academy of Pediatrics, the American Medical Association, the American Psychiatric Association, and the Society for Adolescent Medicine [20].

SUMMARY

Access to quality health care for all is the number one focus area for Healthy People 2010 [22]. There is no question that SBHCs are filling a gap in health care needs for many of our nation's children. Schools with SBHCs are finding that significant physical, mental, and dental health issues are being addressed during the school day, allowing children to remain in school. The mission of SBHCs to contribute to the health of children by providing access to primary health care and preventive health care services is being actualized. Healthy children learn better!

APPENDIX 1

Jose is a 6th grade student sent to the SBHC by his teacher, who is concerned about a persistent cough and frequent episodes of falling asleep in class lately. His grades also are dropping. He meets with the nurse practitioner (NP) and begins to tell his story. His mother left for Puerto Rico 3 weeks ago to care for his ill grandmother and his father is trying to take care of the six children as best he can. Jose is the oldest and is expected to help with his brother and sisters. Jose has asthma but his father has been unable to get his asthma medicine. He says his father yells all the time and Jose says he wants to run away from home. The NP arranges for Jose to get his medicine, talks to his father about support services, and refers Jose to the social worker who will help him to cope with the issues at home.

APPENDIX 2

Serena, a 5th grade student, visited the SBHC when a body piercing done at home became painful and red. She was treated with antibiotics at the SBHC and avoided possible serious consequences of an infection.

APPENDIX 3

Charisse, a 7th grade student, is brought to the SBHC by a friend because she is having difficulty concentrating, cries in the school bathroom, and can't sleep.

The NP learns that Charisse's mother passed away over the summer. She refers her to the social worker and Charisse is able to join a group of students meeting weekly to discuss living with similar losses.

References

[1] World Health Organization, Fifty-sixth World Health Assembly. International Conference on Primary Care, Alma-Ata: twenty-fifth anniversary. Report of the Secretariat. April 24, 2003.

[2] Guernsey BP, Pastore DR. Comprehensive school-based health centers: implementing the model. In: Juszczak L, Fisher M, editors. Health care in schools (Adolescent Medicine, State of the Art Reviews). Philadelphia: Hanley and Belfus, Inc.; 1996. p. 181–96.

[3] Juszczak L, Schlitt J, Odlum M, et al. School-based health centers: national census-school year 2001–2002. Washington (DC): National Assembly on School-based Health Care; 2003.

[4] Hutchins VL, Grason H, Aliza B, et al. Community Access to Child Health (CATCH) in the historical context of community pediatrics. Pediatrics 1999;103(6):1373–83.

[5] Brodeur P. School-based health clinics. In: Isaacs SL, Knickman JR, editors. To improve health and health care 2000: the Robert Wood Johnson anthology. San Francisico (CA): Jossey-Bass; 1999.

[6] Morone JA, Kilbreth EH, Langwell KM. Back to school: a health care strategy for youth. Health Aff 2001;20(1):122–36.

[7] Health Insurance Reform Proposals of the Democratic Presidential Candidates. Available at: http://64.233.167.104/search?q=cache:rBpjomRFqxcJ:www.factcheck.org/UploadedFiles/Ken%2520Thorpe%2520analysis%25209-5-03.doc. Accessed February 21, 2005.

[8] Wold S. School nursing: a framework for practice. St. Louis (MO): The C.V. Mosby Company; 1981.

[9] Lear JG. School-based clinics and adolescent health: past, present and future. In: Juszczak L, Fisher M, editors. Health care in schools (Adolescent Medicine, State of the Art Reviews). Hanley and Belfus, Inc.; 1996. p. 163–80.

[10] Ford L. The school nurse role–a changing concept in preparation and practice. J Sch Health 1970;40(1):21–3.

[11] Igoe JB. The school nurse practitioner. Nurs Outlook 1975;23:381–4.

[12] Friedrich MJ. 25 years of school-based health care. JAMA 1999;281(9):7781–2.

[13] Critical caring on the frontline. Why the need? School-based health centers. Available at: http://www.healthinschools.org/FS/fsneed.html. Accessed February 24, 2005.

[14] Children's Defense Fund. Leave No Child Behind Movement. Available at: http://www.childrensdefense.org/familyincome/childpoverty/default.asp. Accessed February, 21, 2005.

[15] National Center for Health Statistics. Summary health statistics for US children. National Health Interview Survey, 2003. Available at: http://www.cdc.gov/nchs/data/series/sr_10/sr10_221.pdf. Accessed February 28, 2005.

[16] Blum RW, Beuhring T, Wunderlich M, et al. Don't ask, they won't tell: the quality of adolescent health screening in five practice settings. Am J Public Health 1996;86(12):1767–72.

[17] Childstats.gov. America's children 2003. Adolescent mortality. Available at: http://www.childstats.gov/ac2003/indicators.asp?IID=130. Accessed February 27,2005.

[18] Pastore DR, Techow B. Adolescent school-based health care: a description of two sites in their 20th year of service. Mount Sinai J Med 2004;71(3):191–6.

[19] Margins to the Mainstream, Institutionalizing School-based Health Centers. Three states build support for school-based health centers. Available at: http://www.healthinschools.org/sbhcs/papers/conclusion.htm. Accessed March 5,2005.

[20] Flaherty LT, Weist MD, Warner BS. School-based mental health services in the United States: history, current models and needs. Community Ment Health J 1996;32(4):341–52.

[21] The Center for Health and Health Care in Schools. School-based health centers–background. Available at: http://www.healthinschools.org/sbhcs/sbhc.asp. Accessed April 30, 2005.
[22] National Center for Health Statistics. Healthy People 2010. Tracking the nation's health. Available at: http://www.cdc.gov/nchs/about/otheract/hpdata2010/2010fa28.htm. Accessed April 30, 2005.

Nurs Clin N Am 40 (2005) 607–617

NURSING CLINICS
OF NORTH AMERICA

ELSEVIER
SAUNDERS

School of Nursing Sponsorship of a School-Based Health Center: Challenges and Barriers

Judith Scully, PhD, RN, CCHNS, Diana Hackbarth, PhD, RN*

Loyola University Chicago, Niehoff School of Nursing, 6526 North Sheridan Road, Chicago, IL 60626, USA

School-based health centers (SBHCs) are a growing phenomenon in the United States and appear to be an ideal fit for school of nursing (SON) sponsorship. However, nationally only about 6% of existing SBHC are sponsored by either a school of nursing or a school of medicine [1]. Sponsorship of health care in schools is consistent with the mission of university-based SONs, but also presents many challenges. The main mission of a university-based SON is to educate nursing students and support the faculty role of education, practice, research, and service. The goal of a SBHC is to increase access to primary health care, mental health, and dental services, and to provide health education and health promotion interventions to reduce health disparities and enhance the health and ability to learn of the school-aged population. There is an inherent conflict between the faculty role and the direct service role of providing primary health care 12 months a year, 5 days a week, with 24-hour accountability, regardless of a university's academic calendar. The time that it takes for faculty to establish collaborative relationships, write multiple grants to support the SBHC, and provide ongoing management and monitoring of services is also challenging. Assuming responsibility for primary care services for a vulnerable population is a huge responsibility that cannot be taken lightly. However, the authors believe that the benefit to nursing students, faculty, and the profession far outweigh constraints. This article describes the many benefits that can occur when SONs create and maintain a SBHC in their own community. Extensive practical suggestions for how to overcome the barriers that constrain university faculty from developing service-oriented programs in the community are also emphasized.

*Corresponding author. *E-mail address:* dhackba@luc.edu (D. Hackbarth).

0029-6465/05/$ – see front matter
doi:10.1016/j.cnur.2005.07.007

IMPETUS FOR SCHOOLS OF NURSING TO DEVELOP SCHOOL-BASED HEALTH CENTERS

The history of national SBHCs is discussed by Gustafson elsewhere in this issue. In 1995, the Department of Health and Human Services, Health Resources and Services Administration (HRSA) [2] made grant funds available and sponsored national workshops to encourage SONs to develop "nursing practice arrangements" that included the development of SBHCs. In addition to the provision of direct primary health care and preventive services, the goal of these nursing practice arrangements is to increase the primary care workforce by exposing baccalaureate and masters nursing students to primary health care, community health nursing, and traditionally underserved populations. Health science students who are exposed to positive primary care and health promotion experiences in the community are more likely to seek employment in underserved areas and provide culturally sensitive health care. Another goal of the HRSA initiative is to help alleviate the nursing shortage by encouraging young people to seek careers in health care. Funding encourages SONs to partner with schools and community organizations to create innovative programs to showcase nursing as a desirable career option. Finally, the HRSA initiative encourages SONs to collaborate with public health agencies in the areas of education, practice, research, and evaluation as a way to strengthen the public health workforce.

Some SONs that have chosen to develop SBHCs or school-linked health centers have taken advantage of federal HRSA funding. Other SON-sponsored SBHCs have state or local funding. Many SONs use a combination of federal, state, school district, and private foundation funding to support SBHC programs.

BENEFITS OF SCHOOL-BASED HEALTH CENTER SPONSORSHIP FOR SCHOOLS OF NURSING DEMONSTRATING NURSING MODELS OF CARE

There are many benefits for SONs that choose to develop a SBHC. Elementary and secondary schools are ideal community settings to implement a holistic nursing model of care. Although most SBHCs are designed to offer primary health care and many have staff that includes a nurse practitioner or physician's assistant, not all SBHCs operate on a health promotion, disease prevention nursing model. SBHCs sponsored by hospitals or academic medical centers may deliver care in a medical or clinical model. However, almost all SBHCs struggle with balancing the need to provide primary health care services within the health center with the equally compelling need to provide health promotion and education within the school and community. SON sponsorship makes it more likely that a health promotion model will guide care and that nursing interventions will be valued equally with medical care. The authors believe that SON sponsorship of school-based and school-linked health care is the best way to assure that nursing care and advanced practice nurses continue to be valued in schools. Many SBHCs are located in areas that serve many minority children. SON sponsorship of SBHCs can advance the mission of SONs by interesting minority children and youth in considering the profession of nursing as a career option. The United States is confronting the most intense shortage of nursing professionals in its history. By the year 2020, it is estimated that there will be a shortage of 800,000 nurses [3]. Minority groups are under-represented in the nursing workforce. According to the National Sample Survey of Registered Nurses, there are over 2 million nurses in the United States [4]. Of the 2 million nurses, only 4.9% are African American, 3.7% are Asian/Pacific Islander, 2.0% are Hispanic, and 0.5% are Native American/Alaskan Native. One of the best ways to assure that the diverse population of the United States receives culturally competent care is to increase the number of nurses who are from various racial/ethnic backgrounds. In addition, the health care field is one of the best places to have assurance of a job in the years to come [3]. The presence of a SBHC and role modeling of nursing by SBHC staff and SON students can help to inspire young people of color to join the nursing workforce. SON sponsorship of SBHCs is also an ideal way to actualize the mission of hospitals and academic health centers because of opportunities to provide highly regarded direct services for the community. Hospitals and academic health centers are obligated to provide community benefits to maintain their nonprofit status. Forging a partnership with a local SON in sponsoring and maintaining a SBHC is an ideal way to publicly demonstrate the provision of community benefit and maintain nonprofit status.

LABORATORY FOR STUDENT LEARNING

Opportunities for service-learning and clinical practica are abundant in SBHC settings. Undergraduate freshman nursing students can be involved in community experiences such as health fairs and community events, and can pair up with senior students on home visits. For example, home visits can be made to teen mothers to assess their home situations, or to the homes of children excluded from school because of an acute health condition. Sophomore nursing students, who have learned basic nursing skills, can staff booths at health fairs, assist with health screenings, and engage children in health care career exploration. Student nurses can be excellent role models for elementary and high school students. Junior and senior nursing students in their community health, mental health, medical-surgical, obstetrics/gynecology, and pediatric rotations can organize and implement classroom teaching and design health promotion interventions such as exercise groups, smoking prevention, safety, and sexually transmitted infection prevention. Intensive clinical experiences may also be designed for senior undergraduate students who could work one-on-one with a nurse practitioner, health educator, or mental health provider. Registered nurse students seeking a baccalaureate degree can be assigned to the SBHC for a one-semester community health nursing experience. For example, a pair of RN/BSN students can be assigned to organize, supervise, and evaluate a large community health fair or influenza inoculation clinic for the community surrounding the SBHC. The deliverable product at the end of the semester can be a workbook, listing the step-by-step process needed to organize a health fair or inoculation clinic serving 300 to 500 people.

An important advantage of working at a SBHC for undergraduates is that SBHCs often serve ethnically and socially/economically diverse populations. The 2001 to 2002 National Assembly on School-Based Health Care (NASBHC) survey of SBHCs suggests that about one third of the children served are African American, one third are Hispanic, and one third are White, Asian, or other [1]. In addition, many SBHCs are located in urban and rural areas where poverty and lack of access are prevalent. Opportunities to interact and learn from children, parents, and teachers who may have backgrounds different from that of the nursing student can be extremely beneficial. For example, a nursing student presenting a 5-minute presentation on safety and accident prevention at a busy health fair can interact with hundreds of community residents and school-aged children in one day. These experiences can be eye opening when nursing students realize that many families do not own cars, may not have car seats, and that not all children own bicycles. Parental safety concerns may center on protecting their children from violence in the community and not whether the child has a bike helmet. Similarly, undergraduate students assigned to the SBHC for an entire rotation can develop relationships with students who have chronic illness and their parents and learn how culture and socioeconomic status can affect disease management. Students can be guided to focus on the resources and strengths of underserved populations. Working at a SBHC can help to dispel myths and stereotypes so that students begin to recognize the importance of not forcing individuals into categories with certain characteristics [5]. Having experiences in a SBHC helps nursing students think in new ways about resiliency characteristics and risk factors of underserved populations. Talking about culture in the classroom does not always transfer into behaviors until students experience for themselves and appreciate what it means to live in a multicultural society. These opportunities help prepare nursing students to provide culturally competent health care when they embark on their professional careers.

SBHCs are also ideal settings for clinical placements of advanced practice nursing students. If the nursing profession believes that nurse practitioners provide a unique holistic model of primary health care, then graduate students need to be mentored by expert nurse practitioners. Role modeling culturally appropriate nursing interventions is an effective way to prepare advanced practice nursing students to assume roles in the primary health care workforce. A SBHC can serve as a clinical site for family, women's health, and pediatric nurse practitioners. Advanced practice nursing students benefit from exposure to health promotion and risk reduction interventions, and learn how to incorporate resiliency building strategies into nurse practitioner care. In addition, the SBHC affords students the opportunity to observe the importance that SBHC professionals place on students' involvement in their own health care. The SBHC's primary care physician can also serve as a clinical preceptor and role model for collaborative relationships between physicians and nurses. Graduate students are more likely to get a more holistic perspective on primary health care in a nurse-managed SBHC than if they have clinical experiences in physician's offices or hospital clinics, which are likely to operate on a medical model.

FACULTY PRACTICE SITE

SON sponsorship also facilitates maintenance of advanced practice certification for faculty. Many masters and doctoral-prepared faculty actively practice in their specialty area as part of maintaining expertise for their faculty role. Without a dedicated practice site, nursing faculty may find it difficult to preserve clinical expertise because of time constraints. Nursing school sponsorship of a SBHC allows for control of clinical practice times because the university and the SON establish the model of care, staffing pattern, and hours of operation. For example, faculty in women's health can schedule female adolescents for care on days that they are free to provide clinical services. Pediatric faculty can schedule children seeking primary care and meetings with parents of children who have chronic illness on days that they do not have competing teaching responsibilities. Faculty who specialize in mental health can facilitate stress reduction groups on afternoons or evenings set aside for their own clinical practice. Students and faculty can enhance their appreciation of the importance of providing care at times that are convenient to students and families. Faculty who are family nurse practitioners can work with advanced practice students to provide school and sports physical examinations during the summer months and log many hours of clinical practice needed to maintain family nurse practitioner certification. If medical students, residents, and pediatric fellows are also involved in the SBHC, less hectic summer months provide an ideal time for collaboration in the provision of school physicals, immunization, and health promotion activities. Summer day camps for children who have chronic illness, such as diabetes or asthma, may be cosponsored with community agencies and staffed by nursing and medical students and their faculty supervisors. It is the authors' experience that opportunities for creative faculty practice and community service are enhanced when SBHCs partner with community agencies, health departments, hospitals, and academic health centers.

INTERDISCIPLINARY LEARNING

Graduate students in the disciplines of dietetics, health education, psychology, medicine, and social work, and graduate nurses studying informatics and management can benefit from experiences in SBHCs. For example, nursing informatics students can help design and implement management information systems, billing systems, and data collection mechanisms for quality improvement. Other nursing informatics students can evaluate existing management information systems and install the upgrades needed to meet expectations of partners and funders. Graduate nursing students in management practica can be precepted by the SBHC clinical nurse manager and learn the management/leadership skills of vision, collaboration, delegation, empowerment, negotiation, and communication. Medical students can work with the nurse practitioner, health educator, or physician and gain an appreciation for different provider roles and interdisciplinary collaboration. Psychology and social work students could have clinical practica within the SBHC and be mentored by the mental health provider. Dietetic students are a valuable asset and can work one-on-one or with groups of elementary and high school students on issues of good nutrition, weight management, exercise, or eating disorders. Young people who have chronic illnesses such as diabetes or food allergies would especially benefit from interactions with dietetic students. A benefit for all disciplines is the opportunity to learn culturally competent health care delivery in an environment where the philosophy of the setting encourages interdisciplinary collaboration; partnerships between providers and clients; and community participation. The negotiation of positive working relationships between health care providers, school administrators, teachers, and parents is another skill that can be learned.

Site for nursing research

Opportunities for nursing research are also prevalent in SBHCs. Research questions frequently arise from nursing practice. School-aged children and adolescents served by SBHCs often have many health, mental health, and social problems that could be the focus of nursing research. However, research in schools must be handled with the utmost sensitivity. Parents, school administrators, and the community may be extremely wary of the idea of using the SBHC as a research setting and their children as subjects. Children's time spent in the classroom is highly valued and activities that take away classroom time could be perceived as interfering with the mission of the school. The emphasis on testing and meeting federal and state requirements of the No Child Left Behind Act has accentuated this perception. In addition, many elementary and high schools or school districts do not have an Institutional Review Board for the Protection of Human Subjects (IRB) or a mechanism to review research proposals to judge the merits of proposed nursing research.

To conduct research in schools, faculty and doctoral students need to establish a trusting relationship with administrators, teachers, and parents and prove their worth to the school before requesting permission to access students. The responsibility to be well versed in federal regulations governing research on human subjects, Health Insurance Portability and Accountability Act (HIPPA) regulations, and Family Educational Rights and Privacy Act rules is integral to the research role. IRB review can often be sought from the university sponsor of the SBHC. Nurse researchers must be true to their word and uphold the highest standards of honestly and integrity throughout the research process. Sharing the results of research with all stakeholders while maintaining student confidentiality is essential and will go a long way to assure that other nurse researchers will have the opportunity to conduct research in the SBHC in the future. The NASBHC and the Center for Health and Health Care in Schools maintain Web sites that list research and evaluation studies relevant to school-aged children and SBHCs (www.nasbhc.org and www.healthinschools.org, respectively). Priorities for research on the health needs of children and adolescents, and funding opportunities are listed on the Web sites of government agencies, professional associations, and voluntary health organizations concerned with the well-being of children and youth. Experiences in a SBHC can generate ideas for research, and accessing Web sites devoted to school-based health care can aid graduate students and faculty in locating resources and funding for nursing research.

CHALLENGES FOR SCHOOL OF NURSING SPONSORSHIP OF SCHOOL-BASED HEALTH CENTERS

Despite the many benefits of sponsorship of SBHCs, there are challenges and barriers that university administrators and faculty need to consider before they make the commitment to sponsor a SBHC. These challenges are centered on the support or lack of support of university administrators for the establishment and maintenance of direct services in the community; faculty role conflicts; time constraints; and lack of expertise of faculty in terms of developing and managing direct health care services. Other issues relate to the necessity for the university and its faculty representatives to establish ongoing, trusting relationships with community partners. There is nothing worse for the reputation of a university than to initiate programs in disadvantaged communities and then not follow through on commitments.

Commitment from university administration

Deans of SONs must communicate with university administrators to promote understanding of the importance of a SBHC in meeting the mission of the university. Rank and Tenure guidelines should be flexible enough to encompass SBHC implementation as a valuable component of the faculty role. Credit needs to be given to faculty for their huge contribution to the mission of the university and SON if they take on the responsibility for initiating and managing a SBHC in the community.

Deans must also support faculty with the assurance that they will be provided release time for faculty development and management responsibilities. The authors' experience suggests that the lead faculty who develop and manage the SBHC need at least 2 years of 100% release time to initiate the program. Once the SBHC is up and running, 50% release time is needed for grant management and administration of a SBHC. A faculty team approach, with several faculty sharing responsibilities for grant writing and evaluation activities, is also helpful. Funding resources of the SON need to be structured to provide the time and summer salary necessary to assure success. This structuring may mean that faculty usually on a 9-month academic contract receive a 12-month contract to develop and maintain services 52 weeks a year, 5 days per week, with 24/7 responsibility.

The entire faculty of the SON needs to have "buy in" for the SBHC to be successful. Otherwise, faculty may not feel ownership and will be less willing to pitch in when needed or supervise students in a nontraditional SBHC clinical experience. Opportunities must be provided for faculty not directly involved in the initiation of a SBHC to visit the SBHC, interact with staff, and learn about the various opportunities for clinical practice and research. Although a core group of SBHC champions is needed, the commitment of the dean and all faculty is essential for success.

DEVELOPING MANAGEMENT SKILLS

Another important issue is that many nursing faculty members do not initially have the skill set necessary to develop, implement, and maintain a complex organization such as a SBHC. Faculty managing SBHCs need expertise in strategic planning; budgeting; marketing; hiring and evaluating personnel; monitoring day-to-day operations; and evaluation of outcomes. They also need to be familiar with the various regulations that govern health care, employment, and children in schools. This barrier can be overcome by using university-sponsored workshops on personnel management, grant management, and budgeting. Establishing relationships across university departments facilitates smooth management. Use of the university's human resources department for guidelines for recruitment and hiring of staff is essential so that all federal and state employment standards are met. Working with university legal counsel and risk management personnel assures that contracts are properly negotiated and malpractice insurance is in place. Other resources include workshops sponsored by state and national SBHC organizations. In addition, there is a growing number of states and national organizations that publish on-line manuals on designing, implementing, and evaluating SBHC services.

Another important resource for faculty development is consultation with colleagues who have experience in managing school-based health care. Most health care providers involved in school-based health are willing to share their experiences, successes, and failures. Consultation can occur through site visits; networking at state and national coalition meetings; telephone consultations; and joining e-mail list serves.

CULTIVATING TRUST AND MUTUAL SUPPORT

Developing trusting collaborative relationships with elected officials, community partners, advisory boards, administrators, school nurses, teachers, and parents drawn from diverse populations may be an unfamiliar role for some faculty. Faculty enlisted to develop community programs can be drawn from any nursing specialty area, but those who have a background in community health are most likely to have the familiarity and comfort level to work independently in the community. It takes a great deal of time, patience, and tolerance for ambiguity for one to work collaboratively in a community where the university may not be trusted and faculty exert little control. National data on the demographic characteristics of the nursing workforce indicate that 90% of nurses list their race as White. Consequently, faculty of many SONs lack sufficient numbers of people of color. In contrast, about two thirds of the students and families served by SBHCs are either African American or Hispanic, as are many of the employees of the schools in which SBHCs are located. Just as misunderstandings, lack of cultural sensitivity, and tensions sometimes occur between racial groups in the larger society, misunderstanding, cultural faux pas, and tensions can also occur between SON faculty and diverse groups in the school and community. The authors' experience has been that facing the realities of differences and working through them is more productive than denying that these misunderstandings exist. One way to deal with this concern is for SON faculty, SBHC staff, and school and community representatives to jointly participate in formal and informal events to get to know each other better. These opportunities for dialogue can range from something as simple as sharing a meal together to day-long cultural sensitivity workshops. Sometimes mature people have to agree to disagree. Good relationships between people of different socioeconomic, cultural, religious, and ethnic heritages must be worked on and continually refined. This continual growth is consistent with the mission of most universities and SONs and is essential to prepare the nursing workforce of the future to deliver culturally competent care. In addition, individuals benefit from these opportunities to learn and grow with one another.

Differing perspectives between school of nursing faculty, school-based health care providers, and educators in elementary and high schools

Each stakeholder involved in school-based health care has a unique perspective. School administrators operate under educational mandates and see their primary responsibility as education of children. SON faculty priority is the education of students, research, and practice and management of the SBHC. SBHC personnel focus on the provision of primary health care services. School nurses have always dealt with the inherent conflict of being a health care provider in a setting where good health of children is seen as a means to an end and not as an end in itself. SBHC clinicians often experience similar feelings. Clinicians believe that promoting the health of students is the best way to enhance learning. School administrators often perceive attending class as the priority, and receiving health services as secondary.

Given these differing world views, misunderstandings are bound to occur. Tensions may develop over issues of student confidentiality; reproductive services offered in the school; liability; role confusion between the school nurse and the SBHC nurse practitioner; lack of understanding between the school social workers and the SBHC mental health provider; control over the practice of the SBHC; and emergency procedures. Additionally, HIPPA rules preclude sharing of identifiable private health information. In a school setting, the principal may expect to know everything about students and their welfare, but cannot have access to confidential health information.

Schools have a hierarchal governance structure in which superintendents and principals wield a tremendous amount of power. There are established procedures for approval of letters sent home to parents; scheduling of appointments or programs during class or after school; admittance of outside visitors; hours in which the SBHC can operate; and security procedures. Faculty, in contrast, are socialized to believe in academic freedom and are accustomed to independence, setting their own schedules, and being internally accountable with little outside supervision. To be effective, faculty and SBHC staff must learn and work with school procedures and realize that their outside sponsorship makes them guests in the school. One way to effectively deal with differing perspectives is to clearly spell out roles and relationships through legal contracts and letters of agreement, SBHC bylaws, and policies and procedures. The National Association of School Nurses [6] has issued a statement on the importance of collaborative relationships between school nurses and SBHC clinicians and staff. School nurses are natural allies; they can provide valuable insights on negotiating within elementary and high school settings.

However, good interpersonal relationships can go a long way to smooth out differences and solidify trusting relationships.

SUMMARY

The main mission of university-based SONs is the education of nursing students and supporting the faculty role of education, practice, research, and service. The goal of SBHCs is to increase access to primary health care, mental health, and dental services, and to provide health education and health promotion interventions to reduce health disparities and enhance the health and ability to learn of the school-aged population. SON sponsorship of a SBHC is an excellent way to fulfill the mission of a university and an SON. Opportunities for students to have experiences in SBHCs with diverse populations can enhance cultural competence and make it more likely that nursing students will seek careers in the primary health care workforce. SBHC sponsorship facilitates faculty practice and offers many opportunities for creative practice-based research. Barriers to SON sponsorship center around the differing mission of a university and the service mission of a primary care practice site. These barriers can be overcome when trusting collaborative relationships are forged between faculty and university administrators, school personnel, and communities. The authors believe that the benefits far outweigh the barriers and recommend that SON faculty consider SBHC sponsorship as one of the ways to demonstrate the value of a nursing model of care and to ensure that nurses continue to be valued in schools.

References

[1] The National Assembly on School-Based Health Care. School-Based Health Centers National Census School Year 2001–2002. 2002. Available at: www.nasbhc.org. Accessed June 10, 2005.

[2] US Department of Health and Human Services, Health Resources and Services Administration. BHPR, basic nurse education and practice. Available at: www.bhpr.hrsa.gov/nursing/comparison.htm. Accessed June 10, 2005.

[3] Johnson & Johnson. The Campaign for Nursing's Future. Available at: www.discovernursing.org. Accessed June 10, 2005.

[4] Spratley E, Johnson A, Sochalski J, et al. Findings from the National Sample Survey of Registered Nurses. Health Resources and Services Administration. Bureau of Health Professions.

2000. Available at: www.bhpr.hrsa/gov/healthworkforce/reports/rnsurvey. Accessed June 10, 2005.

[5] Zoeller D. Serving special populations. Illinois Department of Human Services, Springfield, IL, Prevention Forum 2005;5(2):1–5.
National Association of School Nurses. The role of the school nurse in school based health centers. Position Statement. Available at: www.nasn.org. 2001.

[6] National Association of School Nurses. The role of the school nurse in a school based health center: position paper, June 1986. Available at: www.nasn.org. Accessed June 10, 2005.

Nurs Clin N Am 40 (2005) 619–636

NURSING CLINICS
OF NORTH AMERICA

Funding, Technical Assistance, and Other Resources for School-Based Health Centers

Deidre M. Washington, MPH, CHES[a],*, Laura C. Brey, MS[b]

[a]National Assembly on School-Based Health Care, 666 11th Street, NW, Suite 735, Washington, DC 20001, USA
[b]National Assembly on School-Based Health Care, 6305 Rushingbrook Drive, Raleigh, NC 27612, USA

In hundreds of communities across the country, health care organizations such as hospitals, community health centers, public health departments, and academic institutions are partnering with public schools to promote the health and academic success of students through school-based health centers (SBHCs). SBHCs enhance the health of the school and its inhabitants by offering direct care to students at risk for poor health and academic outcomes, providing important child and adolescent health expertise to curricular activities and augmenting the school's student support services, which are often stretched thin by limited resources and great demand. The first comprehensive SBHCs originated in Dallas, TX, and St. Paul, MN, in the early 1970s [1]. Since their grassroots inception, SBHCs have grown to become a recognized model for delivering health and mental health services to children and adolescents. The 2001–2002 National SBHC Census survey conducted by the National Assembly on School-Based Health Care (NASBHC) reported 1378 SBHCs in 45 states. Most (39%) were located in high schools, whereas 23% were in elementary schools, 18% were in middle schools, 9% were in elementary–middle schools, 7% were in middle–high schools, and 4% were in K–12 schools. SBHCs are located in diverse communities, with most (62%) in urban areas, 25% in rural settings, and 10% in suburban schools [2]. To facilitate the successful implementation of SBHCs, funding options and technical assistance are needed from various resources. This article identifies the various funding sources and technical assistance opportunities that are available for SBHCs at the national, state, and local level.

*Corresponding author. E-mail address: deidrew@nasbhc.org (D.M. Washington).

0029-6465/05/$ – see front matter
doi:10.1016/j.cnur.2005.07.009

FUNDING OPPORTUNITIES FOR SCHOOL-BASED HEALTH CENTERS

SBHCs represent the coming together of several disciplines under one roof: public health, medicine, mental health, and education. They are most often financed by multiple funding sources that favor their unique clinical opportunities. Fig. 1 illustrates examples of the following funding models for SBHCs: federal grants, state grants, local funding, community partnership contributions, foundations, and patient revenue [3]. Appendix 1 provides electronic funding resources for SBHCs.

Federal grants

Title X of the Public Health Service Act: Family Planning Program

Title X is the only federal program dedicated exclusively to family planning and reproductive health care. Designed to provide access to contraceptive supplies and information with priority given to low-income persons, Title X–supported clinics also provide several preventive health services, such as patient education and counseling; breast and pelvic examinations; and cervical cancer, sexually transmitted disease (STD), and HIV screenings [4].

Although the precise level of support for SBHCs from Title X is unknown, health department–sponsored school health centers may find it an appropriate use of funds to provide pregnancy and STD prevention services and interventions in the school-based primary care settings.

Section 330 of the Public Health Service Act

Section 330 of the Public Health Service Act provides funding to federally qualified health centers (FQHCs). Currently, the authorized categories for FQHCs are community health centers; migrant and rural health centers; and health care for the homeless and public housing residents. Although not an authorized special population category, SBHCs are eligible locations for community health centers and can compete for Section 330 funding if they meet the federal requirements.

Section 330 funding requirements include the following:

- Serve all the residents in their service area without regard to income or insurance status.
- Provide services on a sliding fee scale basis (ie, charges are assessed based on family income).
- Provide service to persons in a designated medically underserved area or serve a medically underserved population.
- Ensure that the board of directors reflects the demographics of the service area and that most of the board consists of consumers of services provided by the center [5,6].

SBHCs that meet FQHC requirements but have not competed successfully for 330 funding or choose not to apply for funding can apply for FQHC Look-Alike status. The difference between FQHCs and FQHC Look-Alikes is that FQHCs receive 330 funding and federal benefits and FQHC Look-Alikes receive FQHC federal benefits but no 330 funding. One benefit of obtaining FQHC Look-Alike status is eligibility for cost-based reimbursement under Medicaid and Medicare. Cost-based reimbursement typically results in higher amounts of revenue for SBHCs that are categorized as FQHC Look-Alikes. The Bureau of Primary Health Care is responsible for the recommendation to the Centers for Medicare and Medicaid Services (CMS) to designate health centers as FQHC Look-Alikes; however, CMS has the final authority. The application for FQHC Look-Alike status can be downloaded at ftp://ftp.hrsa.gov/bphc/docs/2003pins/2003-21.doc. SBHCs can apply for FQHC Look-Alike status and 330 funding simultaneously, but unlike the Section 330 funding application process, the FQHC Look-Alike status application process is noncompetitive [5,6].

The requirement that mandates FQHCs to have a consumer governance board precludes most SBHC sponsoring organizations, including hospitals, academic medicine institutions, and schools, from applying for 330 funding or FQHC Look-Alike status [4]. Currently 76 SBHCs receive an estimated $20 million of the total Section 330 appropriation (approximately $1.6 billion) [4]. SBHCs may also be included as Section 330 grantees under their sponsoring community health center's scope of service. Approximately 300 SBHCs are funded through this arrangement [4].

Most SBHCs do not meet FQHC requirements and are not eligible for Section 330 funding; however, like the federal community health centers, SBHCs need core public health support to be sustained. As of this writing, advocates are seeking a separate authorization for SBHCs and a Medicaid policy that assures adequate compensation for the full scope of service delivered in all SBHCs.

Title VIII Section 831 and Title III Section 330 of the Public Health Service Act: Grow Your Own Health Center Nurse Program

The Bureau of Health Professions administers funds to encourage schools of nursing to develop nursing practice arrangements that can include the development of SBHCs. However, it is important for nursing programs to develop strategies early in the SBHC development process that support sustainability of the health centers. In addition to the provision of direct primary health care and preventive services, the goal of these nursing practice arrangements is to increase the primary care workforce by exposing baccalaureate and masters nursing students to primary health care, community health nursing and traditionally underserved populations.

State grants

Many states allocate several funding sources for SBHCs, including the Title V Maternal and Child Health Block Grant (a federal–state block grant), state general revenue, tobacco settlement money, or any combination of these. These grants represent essential funding streams for many SBHC programs and account for a great part of the growth of SBHCs in the last 20 years [7].

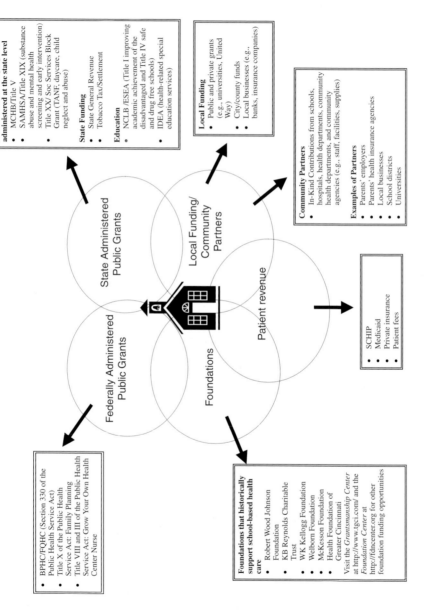

Federal entitlement programs administered at the state level
- MCHB/Title V
- SAMHSA/Title XIX (substance abuse and mental health screening and early intervention)
- Title XX/ Soc Services Block Grant (TANF; daycare, child neglect and abuse)

State Funding
- State General Revenue
- Tobacco Tax/Settlement

Education
- NCLB /ESEA (Title I improving academic achievement of the disadvantaged and Title IV safe and drug free schools)
- IDEA (health-related special education services)

Local Funding
- Public and private grants (e.g., universities, United Way)
- City/county funds
- Local businesses (e.g., banks, insurance companies)

Community Partners
- In-Kind Contributions from schools, hospitals, health departments, community health departments, and community agencies (e.g., staff, facilities, supplies)

Examples of Partners
- Parents' employers
- Parents' health insurance agencies
- Local businesses
- School districts
- Universities

State Administered Public Grants

Local Funding/ Community Partners

Federally Administered Public Grants

Patient revenue

Foundations

- SCHIP
- Medicaid
- Private insurance
- Patient fees

- BPHC/FQHC (Section 330 of the Public Health Service Act)
- Title X of the Public Health Service Act: Family Planning
- Title VIII and III of the Public Health Service Act: Grow Your Own Health Center Nurse

Foundations that historically support school-based health care
- Robert Wood Johnson Foundation
- KB Reynolds Charitable Trust
- WK Kellogg Foundation
- Welborn Foundation
- McKesson Foundation
- Health Foundation of Greater Cincinnati

Visit the *Grantsmanship Center* at http://www.tgci.com/ and the *Foundation Center* at http://fdncenter.org for other foundation funding opportunities

The Maternal and Child Health (MCH) block grant (Title V of the Social Security Act), also known as Title V or MCH block grant, is a federal–state block grant that provides support for state programs focusing on health care for women; children and youth; and families [4]. The MCH block grant authorization includes a "free care" clause that stipulates that no one will be denied care because of inability to pay, which is consistent with the philosophy of SBHCs that often serve indigent, undocumented, and uninsured families. Under Title V, states are also mandated to spend 30% of these funds on children who have special care needs and 30% on primary care and preventive services for children and adolescents [4].

Other examples of currently used and potential state funding sources for SBHCs are listed in Box 1.

New efforts for state funds
As state budgets are increasingly shrinking, SBHC administrators are looking at innovative ways to fill funding gaps. For example, the Michigan SBHCs have maximized their revenue by obtaining a federal Medicaid match to their state general funding. By making the argument to federal and state leaders that SBHCs represent an efficient approach for enrolling students in public insurance plans, providing referrals for specialists, and improving immunization and Early Periodic Screening, Diagnostic, and Treatment (EPSDT) rates, they were able to obtain a Medicaid match of $.56 for every dollar of their $3.7 million state SBHC appropriation. This subsidization represents an additional $2 million in government funds. Medicaid managed care health plans serve as the receiving agent for the Medicaid match dollars, and SBHCs contract with the health plans for services. Per year, each SBHC receives $175,000 and each school-linked center receives $225,000. Other states across the country are exploring this strategy.

Local funding and community partnerships
Many SBHC programs receive strong support from local funding sources. On average, 20% of SBHC funding is from local sources, including public and private grants; in-kind resources from school/community health partners; and county funds [8]. Investments of local sources demonstrate community buy-in to SBHCs. Partnerships with community organizations for in-kind resources (eg, staff, facility, supplies) often serve as a viable funding strategy to supplement state and federal SBHC funding. Examples of creative financing strategies include the formation of partnerships for in-kind and cash resources from

Fig. 1. School-based health center funding models. *Abbreviations:* BPHC, Bureau of Primary Health Care; ESEA, Elementary and Secondary Education Act; FQHC, Federally Qualified Health Center; MCHB, Maternal and Child Health Bureau; NCLB, No Child Left Behind; SAMHSA, Substance Abuse and Mental Health Services Administration; TANF, Temporary Assistance for Needy Families.

Box 1: Examples of currently used and potential state funding sources for school-based health centers

- Temporary Aid to Needy Families (TANF) programs: provide job training and pregnancy prevention
- State General Funds: separate appropriations not tied to federal allocations and requirements; states determine eligibility and program requirements
- Tobacco settlement dollars: although they are time limited and eligibility varies by state, these dollars fund SBHCs in Arizona and New Mexico and nonbillable services in Louisiana
- Tobacco tax dollars: fund nonbillable services, such as smoking prevention programs in North Carolina
- Juvenile Justice programs: have been used to fund services and projects related to incarcerated youth and gang prevention
- Section 504 and special education funds: support health care services for children and adolescents who have individual educational plans
- Department of Education Elementary and Secondary Education Act (ESEA): serves as the basis for No Child Left Behind and funds drug prevention, dropout prevention, after-school risk reduction activities, and mental health activities
- Substance Abuse Prevention and Treatment, Public Health Service Act Title XIX Part B, Subpart II: funds substance abuse and mental health screening and early intervention
- Centers for Disease Control and Prevention, Divisions of HIV/AIDS Prevention

parents' employers, parents' health insurance companies (when SBHCs cannot bill that insurer), local businesses, school districts, banks, universities, and other health and mental health organizations and foundations.

Foundations

Private foundation funding has been an important source of money for SBHC planning, start-up, and special initiatives across the country. Typically, these foundations are nongovernmental, nonprofit organizations with funds (usually from a single source such as an individual, family, or corporation) and programs managed by the foundation's own trustees or directors. Private foundations are established to maintain or aid social, educational, religious, or other charitable activities serving the common welfare, primarily through the making of grants. Depending on their funding source, private foundations are also referred to as corporate or company-sponsored foundations and family foundations [9]. Examples of private foundations that have recently funded SBHC-related activities at the national and local levels include The Robert Wood Johnson Foundation, the W.K. Kellogg Foundation, the McKesson Foundation, the Health Foundation of Greater Cincinnati, the Kate B. Reynolds Charitable Trust, and the Welborn Foundation.

Foundations often restrict their funding to specific causes or activities and to nonprofit organizations located or performing activities in particular states or regions of the country. As a result, foundation funding searches by state and topic are a necessity. Organizations such as the Foundation Center in New York (www.fdncenter.org) and the Grantsmanship Center in California (www.tgci.com) offer online foundation funding databases, searchable by state and topic, for the general public's use at no charge. Private repositories of donor information exist in many cities, and most public libraries have donor and foundation reference materials [10,11].

Patient care revenues

Billing public and commercial insurance

In recent years, SBHCs have experienced increasing political pressures to bill commercial and public insurance programs such as Medicaid and the State Child Health Insurance Program (SCHIP) [12,13]. Most SBHCs (69%) collect revenue for health center visits, predominantly from third-party payers such as Medicaid (68%), SCHIP (43%), and private insurance (45%). Nearly one in four SBHCs directly assess fees from the student or family [2]. In a national survey, SBHCs reported that patient revenue accounted for 12% of their total budget [13]. Successful billing for patient revenue requires a billing infrastructure and technical assistance [14]. Without an appropriate infrastructure, collecting patient revenue can strain the SBHC's already limited administrative capacity.

Medicaid and Medicaid managed care

SBHCs can be a partner in states' efforts to improve access to health and mental health care for hard-to-reach and poorly served children and adolescents. As SBHCs have begun to seek diverse funding streams, Medicaid has emerged as an integral component of the SBHC funding portfolio. The ability of SBHCs to use Medicaid as a significant funding source is partly determined by the volume of SBHC users that are enrolled in Medicaid. Because they are strategically located in underserved communities, SBHCs provide care for a disproportionately larger population of publicly insured patients [15]. Data collected by the National Assembly shows that Medicaid reimbursement is the largest source of nongrant patient revenue for SBHCs [13]. State policies on Medicaid reimbursement for school-based health services differ greatly with respect to fiscal support; billing procedures and structures; and requirements for provider credentials [16]. As Medicaid reimbursement becomes an important strategy for sustaining SBHCs, collaboration among SBHCs; state leadership from public health departments; and Medicaid agencies to address reimbursement barriers is critical. For example, in Illinois, the state provides resources to help SBHC staff develop enrollment and billing expertise. States can also designate SBHCs as Medicaid providers. Long-term inclusion of SBHCs as providers in the Medicaid health care system should be promoted by the presence of SBHC representatives at the bargaining table as health care polices are developed.

Many state Medicaid agencies have adopted managed care approaches to organizing, delivering, and financing Medicaid services; however, SBHCs have had varying degrees of success in becoming part of these managed care systems. Some barriers to success in the relationship between SBHCs and managed care are: (1) families that have children in more than one school cannot use a single provider; (2) SBHCs and their community partner must provide 24-hour, 7-day-per-week health care coverage for patients; and (3) the volume of potential enrollees in a school setting is not sufficient to sustain a reasonable risk pool for primary care.

Although many SBHCs report that working with managed care is burdensome and results in significantly less revenue than was generated from Medicaid before managed care, the relationship to the community health care system is still perceived as important. Some states (eg, Connecticut, Rhode Island) have been designated by the state Medicaid agencies as essential community providers or required partners with managed care. This designation has been helpful in building relationships between SBHCs and managed care entities. Other state Medicaid agencies have created managed care "carve outs" (ie, allocated money) for center services (eg, Illinois, New York, Maryland), which have sustained access to Medicaid revenues while long-term solutions to help SBHCs become part of the network for managed care providers can be worked out [12,17].

TECHNICAL ASSISTANCE OPPORTUNITIES FOR SCHOOL-BASED HEALTH CENTERS

As SBHC programs implement creative funding strategies to sustain and expand SBHC services, the need for technical assistance at the national and state level increases. Technical assistance for SBHCs is offered primarily at the national level by trade and membership organizations. State offices and SBHC associations also offer state-specific resources and technical assistance. Several states have created ongoing activities to assist SBHC programs with data collection and evaluation, billing, and managed care negotiations [1].

National technical assistance and resources

Since its inception in 1995, the National Assembly on School-Based Health Care (NASBHC), a nonprofit member organization, has become the national voice and technical assistance provider for SBHCs across the country. NASBHC offers a continuum of professional development activities and resources, including individual SBHC technical assistance, group workshops, continuing education activities, an annual SBHC convention offering over 60 workshops, and a customized web site to provide resources on several topics related to school-based health care. Primary topic areas for NASBHC technical assistance and resources are patient care; SBHC Operations; evaluation and quality; and advocacy/public policy. Fig. 2 shows the dissemination strategies NASBHC employs to provide technical assistance and resources. Descriptions of NASBHC's resources and trainings are listed in Box 2.

Sustainable funding (patient revenue and advocating for public health dollars)

As federal and state budgets tighten, technical assistance and training on billing for services and building advocacy capacity are becoming an increasing need. Data from NASBHC indicate that the SBHC field considers obtaining funding

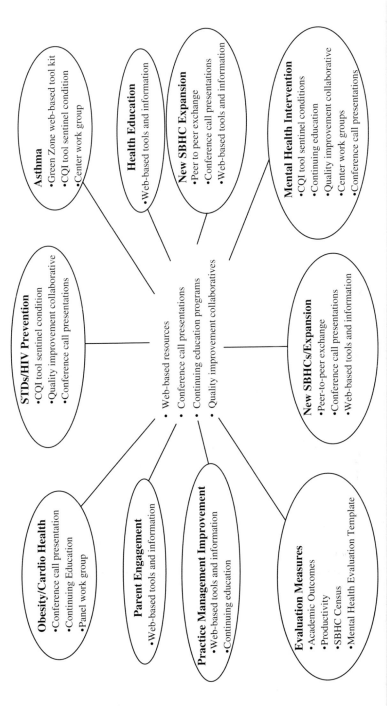

Fig. 2. National assembly' trainings, tools, and resources for SBHCs. *Abbreviation:* CQI, Continuous Quality Improvement.

Box 2: Descriptions of the National Assembly on School-Based Health Care's resources and trainings

Patient care

- Obesity: state-based trainings and online resources
- Mental health: quality improvement initiative that provides trainings and technical assistance to increase evidence-based practice in mental health for SBHC providers
- Parental engagement: resources for SBHCs on how to develop programs that increase parental engagement
- Health education: online resource, offering an array of health education materials for students in English and Spanish
- STD/HIV prevention: quality improvement program that provides training in group and individual prevention modalities to prevent STD/HIV in adolescents
- Asthma: tool kit with resources for school personal, parents, students, and clinicians on asthma care management
- Comprehensive risk assessment: regional and local trainings on the implementation of risk assessments

School-based health center operations

- SBHC general operations: site technical assistance and workshops on SBHC startup; medical coding; developing policies and procedures; and implementing effective systems
- Practice management: quality improvement initiative that provides intensive technical assistance on best practices in SBHC operations

Evaluation and quality

- Academic outcomes: recommendations for SBHC professionals on how to measure academic outcomes related to school-based health care
- Productivity: workshops and tools for measuring provider productivity in SBHCs
- Census: online and hard copy resource with SBHC data
- Mental health evaluation template: online tool for measuring quality indicators in SBHC mental health programs
- Continuous quality improvement tool: hard copy and data application measurement tool for SBHC services

Advocacy and public policy

- Communications tools: resources for developing media relations and communication messages
- Organizational development: technical assistance on leadership development
- Community mobilization: workshops and technical assistance on grassroots advocacy and organizing communities
- Advocacy: tools and resources for communicating with legislators
- Funding: resources and technical assistance on grant writing and funding opportunities

and billing for services as critical areas where resources and technical assistance are needed [18]. Nationally, SBHC programs have reported that in order for them to be successful at billing for services, they need technical assistance and resources in the following areas:

- Management information systems that collect encounter and billing data to eliminate the double entry required to maintain two separate systems
- Services of dedicated billing specialist staff to augment the already busy clinicians and front desk staff
- Training and support for providers on medical coding and documentation [14]

Although billing for services can be a cumbersome task without the proper support and infrastructure, SBHC programs across the country have been successful at incorporating a billing structure, streamlining the billing process, and increasing patient revenue.

Dollars from patient revenue can provide substantial support for SBHC services; however, the supposition that SBHCs can be made financially stable through billing is not practical for most SBHCs. Stable public health funding is needed to sustain SBHCs. To help build capacity for states to obtain public health dollars for SBHCs, NASBHC provides training and technical assistance on grassroots lobbying, community mobilization, legislative advocacy, media communication, and marketing techniques. Using these strategies, SBHC advocates can work to increase public support for SBHCs.

Technical assistance and Medicaid

Public insurance programs such as Medicaid are a critical resource for SBHCs; however, the billing and collections process has been problematic in some SBHC settings. Based on informational sessions conducted by NASBHC with key stakeholders (providers and administrators), the following obstacles were noted regarding Medicaid billing [12]:

- Medicaid's free care policy requiring health centers to bill non-Medicaid clients is burdensome. Full-time billing and collections staff are needed to collect fees, insurance copays, and deductibles, and to track insurance status of users.
- Billing of health plans and commercial insurers that results in an "explanation of benefits" being forwarded to the client's home is considered a breach of confidentiality. As a result, providers are reluctant to bill for potentially confidential services.
- Uninsured children and adolescents are a significant problem in some communities, especially where immigrant populations are not eligible or families simply do not want to be on public assistance.
- School-based health care providers have difficulty acquiring accurate and updated insurance information from students.
- State Medicaid/SCHIP services and provider eligibility may preclude revenue recovery for certain school-based providers (eg, nurse practitioners, clinical social workers) or services (eg, preventive mental health and counseling, including individual, family, and group; risk assessment; health education; self-management of chronic issues)

• Medicaid reimbursement is often not reinvested back into the school health services, reducing incentives for programs to invest in billing capacity [12].

NASBHC has created tools and resources in the area of practice management improvement that provide useful information and strategies for increasing patient revenue from Medicaid and commercial insurers. Some of these strategies include improved documentation and coding; redesign and routine updating of provider encounter forms; and productivity monitoring and benchmarking.

Other national professional organizations, such as the Society for Adolescent Medicine, the National Association of Pediatric Nurse Practitioners, the National Association of Community Health Centers, and the American School Health Association, offer special interest groups in the area of school-based health care for networking and problem solving among their membership. Additionally, organizations such as The Center for Health and Health Care in Schools at the George Washington University and The Center for School Mental Health Assistance at the University of Maryland offer resources and trainings specific to the school-based health care field. Many of these organizations have been involved in the school-based health care movement since its inception, and work collaboratively with NASBHC. Appendix 2 provides web site addresses for the above national organizations.

State technical assistance, training, and resources

State associations

State SBHC associations provide state-specific technical assistance and resources for SBHCs. Nationally there are 20 state SBHC associations. Results from a state SBHC association assessment demonstrate that these organizations are providing an array of services to SBHCs. These services include advocacy; functioning as an information center and clearinghouse; and providing technical assistance, opportunities for member networking, continuing education, grant/funding alerts, advocacy alerts, and association news updates [19]. In April 2004, 9 of the 20 state associations received funding to support broad-based advocacy targeted at increasing funding for SBHCs. As a result, the state associations have strengthened their capacity to provide technical assistance and resources on advocacy, grassroots mobilization, and communication strategies. Table 1 illustrates the resources that each state association provides and Appendix 3 provides contact information for each state SBHC association.

State health departments and primary care associations

State health departments and primary care associations also serve as state-specific resources for SBHCs across the country. Many state departments of health provide funding support, tools, and training workshops for SBHCs. Some state primary care associations also provide in-kind support (eg, facilities and staff), technical assistance, and advocacy support for SBHCs. In Massachusetts, Michigan, West Virginia, and Illinois, the state primary care associations have close relationships with the SBHCs.

Table 1

State school-based health care associations member services

Member services	AZ	CA	CO	CT	FL	IL	KY	LA	MA	MD	ME	MI	NC	NM	NY	OH	OR	TX	WV	No.	%
Information/clearinghouse	✓	✓	✓	✓	✓	✓	✓						✓		✓	✓			✓	11	58%
Technical assistance	✓	✓	✓	✓	✓	✓	✓				✓	✓	✓		✓	✓			✓	12	63%
Continuing education	✓	✓	✓	✓	✓				✓			✓	✓			✓	✓	✓	✓	12	63%
Grant/funding alerts	✓	✓	✓	✓	✓	✓	✓	✓	✓	✓		✓	✓	✓	✓	✓	✓		✓	18	95%
Advocacy alerts		✓	✓	✓	✓	✓	✓	✓	✓	✓	✓	✓	✓	✓	✓	✓	✓	✓	✓	18	95%
Information and referral	✓	✓	✓	✓	✓	✓	✓	✓	✓		✓	✓	✓	✓		✓	✓			15	79%
Association news/updates	✓	✓	✓	✓	✓	✓	✓	✓	✓	✓	✓	✓	✓	✓	✓	✓	✓		✓	18	95%

Other categories states added: advocacy and opportunities for member networking.

Courtesy of the National Assembly on School-Based Health Care, Washington DC, as of March 2004.

SUMMARY

SBHCs need federal policies and state/local funding that will sustain and develop the school-based health care field. The most stable funding strategies for SBHCs employ diverse funding sources, including federal grants, state grants, local funding, foundation grants, patient revenue, and collaborative partnerships. Common funding sources for SBHCs include Section 330 of the Public Health Service Act, Title X of the Public Health Service Act: Family Planning Program (federal); the Maternal and Child Health Block Grant (Title V of the Social Security Act); General Revenue Funds (state); county and city health departments; private foundations; Medicaid and SCHIP (patient revenue); and in-kind staff and facilities (community partnerships).

SBHCs' increased focus on funding to sustain and expand services has created a greater need for technical assistance and training at the national and state level. National professional organizations, state SBHC associations, state health departments, and primary care associations offer various resources and technical assistance opportunities specific to school-based health care. For SBHCs to remain viable entities in the health care system, they should consider diversifying funding support and forming relationships with organizations that offer school-based health care–specific technical assistance and resources.

APPENDIX 1

Resources for Funding SBHC Activities

Governmental Resources	Web site
Centers for Disease Control and Prevention (CDC), National Center for Chronic Disease Prevention and Health Promotion, (NCCDPHP), Division of Adolescent and School Health (DASH), Preventive Health Services Block Grant (PHSBG)	www.cdc.gov/nccdphp www.cdc.gov/healthyyouth/partners/index.htm www.cdc.gov/healthyyouth/funding/index.htm www.federalgrantswire.com/preventive_health_and_health_services_block_grant.html
Centers for Medicare and Medicaid (CMS), Medicaid	www.cms.hhs.gov/medicaid/
Centers for Medicare and Medicaid (CMS), State Child Health Insurance Program (SCHIP)	www.cms.hhs.gov/schip/
Department of Health and Human Services (DHHS), Administration for Children and Families (ACF), Office of Family Assistance (OFA), Temporary Assistance for Needy Families (TANF)	www.acf.dhhs.gov/programs/ofa/ www.policyalmanac.org/social_welfare/archive/ssbg.shtml
Department of Health and Human Services (DHHS), Office of Public Health and Science (OPHS), Office of Population Affairs (OPA), Office of Family Planning (OFP), Title X of the Public Health Service Act	www.opa.osophs.dhhs.gov/titlex/ofp.html

No Child Left Behind (NCLB), Elementary and Secondary Education Act (ESEA), Title I, Part A – Improving the Academic Achievement of the Disadvantaged	www.ed.gov/policy/elsec/leg/esea02/pg1.html
No Child Left Behind (NCLB), Elementary and Secondary Education Act (ESEA), Title IV, Part A – Safe and Drug Free Schools	www.ed.gov/policy/elsec/leg/esea02/pg51.html
Health Resources and Services Administration (HRSA), Bureau of Primary Health Care (BPHC), Section 330/FQHC	www.bphc.hrsa.gov/Grants/Default.htm
Health Resources and Services Administration (HRSA), Center for Health Care Financing and Managed Care - Medicaid Managed Care	www.hrsa.gov/financemc/
Health Resources and Services Administration (HRSA), Maternal and Child Health Bureau (MCHB), Maternal and Child Health Services Block Grant (MCHSBG), Bureau of Health Professions	www.mchb.hrsa.gov/grants/default.htm www.federalgrantswire.com/maternal_and_child_health_services_block_grant_to_the_states.html http://www.hrsa.gov/grants/preview/professions.htm
Individuals with Disabilities Education Improvement Act of 2004 (IDEA)	www.ed.gov/policy/speced/guid/idea/idea2004.html www.ed.gov/parents/needs/speced/resources.html www.ed.gov/about/offices/list/osers/osep/index.html
Substance Abuse and Mental Health Services Administration (SAMHSA), National Mental Health Information Center, Mental Health Block Grant (MHBG)	www.mentalhealth.samhsa.gov/cmhs/Stateplanning/about.asp
Substance Abuse and Mental Health Services Administration (SAMHSA), Substance Abuse Prevention and Treatment, Public Health Service Act Title XIX Part B, Subpart II (substance abuse and mental health screening and early intervention)	www.samhsa.gov/index.aspx
Social Services Block Grant (SSBG), Title XX of the Social Security Act	www.policyalmanac.org/social_welfare/archive/ssbg.shtml
Foundation Resources	
The Foundation Center	www.fdncenter.org
The Grantsmanship Center	www.tgci.com

APPENDIX 2

National organizations with special interest groups or technical assistance/resources for School-based health centers

Name of organization	Web site
National Assembly on School-Based Health Care	www.nasbhc.org
Society for Adolescent Medicine	www.adolescenthealth.org/
National Association of Pediatric Nurse Practitioners	www.napnap.org/index_home.cfm/
National Association of Community Health Centers	http://www.nachc.com/
American School Health Association	www.ashaweb.org
Center for Health and Health Care in Schools	www.healthinschools.org/home.asp
Center for School Mental Health Assistance	http://csmha.umaryland.edu/

APPENDIX 3

State school-based health center associations

Association and Web site (if available)	Contact
Arizona School-Based Health Care Council www.azschoolhealthcouncil.org	James Washington jwashington@abrazohealth.com
California School Health Centers Association http://www.schoolhealthcenters.org	Serena Clayton sclayton@schoolhealthcenters.org
Colorado Association for School-Based Health Care http://www.casbhc.org	Barbara Ford ford@casbhc.org
Connecticut Association of School-Based Health Centers	Melanie Bonjour m.bonjour@ci.danbury.ct.us
District of Columbia Assembly on School Based Health Care	Jennifer Leonard JLeonard@ChildworksPLLC.com
Florida Coalition of School-Based Health Centers	Patricia Stauffer PStauffer@med.miami.edu
Illinois Coalition for School Health Centers http://www.ilmaternal.org/ICSHC_Home.htm	Karen Berg kberg@ilmaternal.org
Kentucky School Based Health Center Collaborative http://www.kychildnow.org/sbhc/	John Webb johnwebb@kychildnow.org
Louisiana Assembly on School-Based Health Care www.lasbhc.org/	Charles Peters capetersjr@yahoo.com
Maine School-Based Health Care Assembly http://www.mainechildrensalliance.org/ am/publish/article_33.shtml	Craig Robinson craighrobinson@yahoo.com
Maryland Assembly on School-Based Health Care www.masbhc.org/	Donna Behrens dbehrens@masbhc.org
Massachusetts Coalition of School-Based Health Centers http://www.mcsbhc.org/	Ernia Hughes ehughes.1@worldnet.att.net
School-Based Community Health Alliance of Michigan http://www.scha-mi.org/	Debbie Brinson dbrinson@scha-mi.org
New Mexico Assembly of School-Based Health Care http://www.nmassembly.org/	Howard Spiegelman hspiegelman@comcast.net
New York Coalition for School-Based Primary Care	Shirley Gordon Gordon@acmenet.net
North Carolina Association of School-Based and Linked Health Centers	Constance N. Parker ConnieParker@whatswhat.org

Ohio School-Based Health Care Association	Barbara Wise
	blwise@health-partners.org
Oregon School-Based Health Care Network	Debbie Kaufman
http://www.osbhcn.org/	debbie@cffo.org
Texas Association of School-Based Health	Retta Knox
Centers http://www.tasbhc.org/	retta.knox@region16.net
West Virginia Assembly of School-Based	Becky King
Health Centers http://www.wvsbha.org	bk517@attglobal.net

As of June 2005.

References

[1] Schlitt J, Rickett KD, Montgomery LL, et al. State initiatives to support school-based health centers: A national survey. J Adolesc Health 1995;17(2):68–76.

[2] Juszczak L, Schlitt J, Odulum M, et al. School-based health center national census, school year 2001–02. Washington (DC): National Assembly on School-Based Health Care; 2003.

[3] National Assembly on School-Based Health Care. A brief look at funding models. Available at: www.nasbhc.org/TAT/AZ%20Finance%20Session.pdf. Accessed February 12, 2005.

[4] Schlitt J. Assessing national opportunities to sustain school-based health centers. Washington (DC): National Assembly on School-Based Health Care; 2005.

[5] US Department of Health and Human Services, Bureau of Primary Health Care. Available at: http://bphc.hrsa.gov/chc/CHCInitiatives/fqhc_lookalike.asp. Accessed June 22, 2005.

[6] US Department of Health and Human Services' Rural Initiative. The Rural Assistance Center (RAC). Available at: http://www.raconline.org/info_guides/clinics/fqhcfaq.php#whatis. Accessed June 22, 2005.

[7] Lear J. School-based health centers: a road less traveled. Arch Pediatr Adolesc Med 2003;157:118–9.

[8] Costin D, Schlitt J. School-based health center finance and revenue study data; June 2002. Available at: http://www.nasbhc.org/APP/Finance_Survey_Overview2.htm. Accessed February 10, 2005.

[9] The Foundation Center. The Foundation Center's user-friendly guide to funding research and resources. Available at: http://fdncenter.org/learn/ufg/ufg_gloss1.html. Accessed June 22, 2005.

[10] The Foundation Center. Finding funders, Web sites of private foundations, private foundation search. Available at: http://fdncenter.org/funders/grantmaker/gws_priv/priv.html. Accessed June 22, 2005.

[11] The Grantsmanship Center. Funding resources. Available at: http://www.tgci.com/funding/resources.asp. Accessed June 25, 2005.

[12] National Assembly on School-Based Health Care. Partners in access: school-based health centers and Medicaid. Washington (DC): National Assembly on School-Based Health Care; 2001.

[13] National Assembly on School-Based Health Care. School-based health center third-party billing policies and systems: NASBHC convenes a workgroup. January 2002. Available at: http://www.nasbhc.org/TAT/work%20group%20summary%202.0%20layout.pdf. Accessed February 10, 2005.

[14] National Assembly on School-Based Health Care. School-based health centers, to bill or not to bill. Available at: http://www.nasbhc.org/TAT/To_Bill_or_Not_to_Bill.htm. Accessed January 10, 2005.

[15] National Assembly on School-Based Health Care. Issue brief, Medicaid reimbursement in school-based health centers: state association and provider perspectives. June 2000. Available at: http://www.nasbhc.org/Membership/Publications/ci2.pdf. Accessed January 15, 2005.

[16] Lear JG, Montgomery LL, Schlitt J, et al. Key issues affecting school-based health centers and Medicaid. J Sch Health 1996;66(3):83–8.

[17] National Assembly on School-Based Health Care. Issue brief, critical issues in school-based health center financing. Washington, DC: September 1999. Available at: http://www.nasbhc.org/Membership/Publications/ci3.pdf. Accessed January 11, 2005.

[18] National Assembly on School-Based Health Care. NASBHC strategic plan survey. Washington (DC): National Assembly on School-Based Health Care; 2005.

[19] National Assembly on School-Based Health Care. State school-based health center association assessment. Washington (DC): National Assembly on School-Based Health Care; 2005.

Nurs Clin N Am 40 (2005) 637–647

NURSING CLINICS
OF NORTH AMERICA

ELSEVIER
SAUNDERS

Cultural Aspects of Working with Students Enrolled in a School-Based Health Center

Susan M. Murray, RN, MPH

The Health Center at Roosevelt High School, Room 166, 3436 West Wilson, Chicago, IL 60625, USA

CULTURE IN SCHOOL-BASED HEALTH CENTERS

School-based health centers (SBHCs) are known to increase access to preventive quality health services to the underserved population of children and adolescents [1]. Typically, SBHCs are located in culturally diverse communities with a high prevalence of low-income families who are uninsured or underinsured. Students attending the schools where SBHCs are located reflect the diversity of their communities. As our nation becomes more culturally diverse, so does the student populations that are served in SBHCs.

A multifaceted approach is required to understand the concept of culture for youth populations. There are several examples of cultural components to consider. The culture of adolescence may include unique language, music, and behavioral trends (eg, experimenting with drugs or alcohol, dieting behavior). The culture of poverty may impact school attendance, eating habits, or vocational plans. The culture of gangs may impact individual behavior and the ability to establish the SBHC as a safe place for youth to seek services. The culture of gay/lesbian/bisexual/transgendered youth may lead to isolation of the individual or conversely result in acting-out behavior. For purposes of this article, *culture* will be defined as the thoughts, communications, actions, customs, beliefs, values, and institutions of a racial, ethnic, religious, or social group [2]. Culture is learned and ever changing.

Acculturation of youth to most culture is a process that can impact the care provided in SBHCs. *Acculturation* is defined as the change that occurs when two different groups come into contact. In general, the group with the least power is forced to change most but can retain distinctive cultural traits [3]. The ability to learn English to achieve success in school or to adopt dietary changes (eg, the high-sugar, high-fat, fast food American diet) may affect the dynamics of power within a young person's family and his health and health-seeking behaviors.

E-mail address: smurray@schosp.org

0029-6465/05/$ – see front matter
doi:10.1016/j.cnur.2005.07.003

CULTURAL DIVERSITY IN SCHOOL-BASED HEALTH CENTERS

According to the National Assembly on School-Based Health Care (NASBHC) Census 2001–2002, the racial/ethnic breakdown of the population served in SBHCs throughout the nation is 33% African American, 32% White, 29% Hispanic/Latino, 4% Asian, 1% Native American, and 1% other [4]. The US Census Bureau has estimated that by the year 2015, the population between 5 and 19 years of age will increase by 10% and the Asian/Pacific Islander and Hispanic groups within this age group will increase by 67% and 69%, respectively [5,6]. Results of a survey of 50 SBHCs from 24 states by the Center for Health and Health Care in Schools in 2004 shows the racial/ethnic diversity of the respondents, who were service providers or administrators, as 72% white, 14% African American, 8% Native American, 4% Hispanic/Latino, and 4% Asian or Pacific Islander [7]. Although these data are not all-inclusive and include SBHC staff who do not provide direct services, the diversity profile of staff to users is imbalanced: 28% of staff belong to a racial minority as compared with 68% of the students. This disparity poses a challenge to the provision of culturally effective health care in the SBHC setting.

SCHOOL-BASED HEALTH CENTER CHALLENGES

According to the NASBHC survey, the most frequent barriers identified by the administrators and clinicians who responded to the survey were language; differing attitudes toward behavioral or mental health issues; trust in the provider by patient or patient's family; and differing attitudes toward Western medicine [7]. Respondents also named the leading challenges to addressing cross-cultural issues as identifying barriers, overcoming financial barriers, and finding staff who represent or are knowledgeable about racial/ethnic groups represented in school [7].

It is well documented that racial/ethnic minorities experience disparities in health services in the United States health care system as compared with their white counterparts [8]. Multiple studies show that health care providers sometimes provide a lower quality care to patients who are from nondominant or minority cultures. Three studies of the school-age population show ethnic differences in vision screening, receipt of prescriptive medications, and treatments. Specifically, Latinos or African American children received fewer vision screenings, prescriptions, and home nebulizer treatments after hospital discharge than white children [9–11].

A 2002 Institute of Medicine report provides further evidence of ethnic differences in health care. The report notes that racial and ethnic minorities receive lower quality care than whites even when insurance status and ability to pay for care are the same. In addition, the report suggested that one of the many reasons for unequal treatment may be the bias, prejudice, and stereotyping on the part of the health care provider. Most distressing is the finding that there is "considerable empirical evidence that even well-intentioned whites who are not overtly biased and who do not believe that they are prejudiced typically demonstrate unconscious implicit negative racial attitudes and stereotypes." The report concludes that it is reasonable to assume that health care providers find prejudice morally wrong and at odds with their professional values and may not recognize manifestations in their own behavior. Research suggests that providers' diagnostic and treatment decisions and their feelings about patients are influenced by the patient's race or ethnicity [12].

The Commission to End Health Care Disparities was developed in response to the identification of these inequalities, specifically the notion that some of the disparity may be the result of poor information and incorrect perceptions on the part of health care providers. In January 2005, three major medical societies and 30 member organizations announced a major initiative "to close the gaps in health care that are based on race and culture" [13]. The Commission to End Health Care Disparities states it will work to raise provider awareness; improve data gathering; increase education and training; and promote workforce diversity [13].

Although more attention is currently focused on the issue of ethnic disparity in health care, the need to provide culturally effective health care is an implicit assumption in the high-quality services SBHCs strive to provide. As part of a larger health care delivery system, SBHCs need to develop a plan to provide culturally and linguistically appropriate services that are respectful of and responsive to cultural and linguistic needs [14]. It is crucial to the development of such a plan to understand that (1) no recipe or formula exists for creating cultural competence, (2) the individual provider and larger system must be involved in the process, and (3) the creation of cultural competence is a continually evolving process [15,16].

As it relates to SBHCs, cultural competence

- Can be a set of congruent behaviors, attitudes, and policies that come together in a system or agency or among professionals and enables that system or agency or those professionals to work effectively in cross-cultural situations [2]
- Describes practices that promote effective cross-cultural communication, responsiveness, and understanding of the diverse issues that accompany any culture [7]
- Is defined simply as the level of knowledge-based skills required to provide effective clinical care to patients from a particular ethnic or racial group [14]

Cultural sensitivity, on the other hand, is the ability to be appropriately responsive to the attitudes, feelings, or circumstances of groups of people that share a common and distinctive racial, national, religious, linguistic, or cultural heritage [17].

MODELS OF CULTURAL COMPETENCE

Numerous models of cultural competence exist. Two models relevant to SBHCs are outlined below.

The first model of cultural competence is Campinha-Bacote's [16] *The Process of Cultural Competence in the Delivery of Healthcare Services*. It defines cultural competence as "the process in which the health care professional continually strives to achieve the ability and availability to effectively work within the cultural context of a client" [16]. The model includes five constructs, as follows:

Cultural awareness is defined as the process of conducting self-examination of one's own biases toward other cultures and the in-depth exploration of one's cultural and professional background.

Cultural knowledge is defined as the process in which the health care professional seeks and obtains a sound information base regarding the worldviews of different cultural and ethnic groups.

Cultural skill is defined as the ability to conduct a cultural assessment to collect relevant cultural data regarding the client's presenting problem and to accurately conduct a culturally based physical examination.

Cultural encounters is the process that encourages the health care professional to directly engage in face-to-face cultural interactions and other encounters with clients from culturally diverse backgrounds to modify existing beliefs about a cultural group and prevent possible stereotyping.

Cultural desire is the motivation of the health care professional to "want to" engage in the process of becoming culturally aware, knowledgeable, and skillful and seek cultural encounters, instead of "have to."

In addition, Campinha-Bacote challenges health care professionals to continuously ask themselves "have I 'ASKED' myself the right questions?":

Awareness: am I aware of my biases and prejudices toward other cultural groups, and racism in health care?

Skills: do I have the skill for conducting a cultural assessment?

Knowledge: am I knowledgeable about worldviews of different cultural and ethnic groups, and educated in the field of biocultural ecology?

Encounters: do I seek face-to-face and other types of interactions with the individuals who are different from myself?

Desire: do I really "want to" become culturally competent? [16]

A second model of cultural competence is Flores' [19] Achieving Cultural Competence in Health Care. This model of cultural competency focuses on the Latino culture but can be used to guide providers in interactions with any cultural group. The model consists of five components with accompanying practical solutions, identified in Box 1.

PRACTICE RECOMMENDATIONS

Practice recommendations that may prove helpful in building culturally competent services in an SBHC include the provision of educational opportunities for staff, students, and their families and the use of operational tools to standardize care and measure client satisfaction. Another strategy to increase cultural diversity in the health care workforce is engaging in outreach with students to promote entry into health careers as a potential career choice after graduation. This section presents practical suggestions and several resources that address practice recommendations and student strategies.

Box 1: Flores' Achieving Cultural Competence in Health Care model

Normative culture values

Identify those that affect care

Accommodate for these in clinical encounters

Language issues

Use interpreter services unless fluent in patient's primary language

Follow guidelines for effective interpreter use

Encourage efforts to increase foreign language skills of staff and English skills of patients who have limited English proficiency

Folk illnesses

Recognize those that may affect clinical care

Suggest alternatives to harmful folk remedies

Accommodate for these in nonjudgmental manner during clinical encounter

Integrate these into biomedical treatment plan whenever possible

Patient/parent beliefs

Identify those that may affect clinical care

Suggest alternatives to harmful home remedies

Carefully explain cause and treatment rationale for given biomedical condition

Provider practices

Maintain vigilance for ethnic disparities in screening, prescriptions, procedures, and outcomes

When disparities occur, determine source of problems and address practices that might be responsible [18,19]

Staff training/education

The delivery of culturally effective health care includes having a provider who is culturally competent; does not stereotype the patient's needs; provides a balance between the patient's needs and expectations in the relationship; and respects those needs and expectations. Recommendations to other school health centers from the respondents in the NASBHC survey include [7]:

- Listen to students and their families carefully. Do not make assumptions.
- Eliminate language barriers whenever possible. Seek materials written in other languages. Use interpreters to overcome barriers. Learn the language whenever possible.
- Provide cultural competence workshops for staff. Use members of the school's community if possible.
- Learn about the school's diverse populations. Do not categorize by race and language only.
- Hire staff to reflect the diversity of the school's community.

- Form relationships with members of the community. Get to know the families and involve them in health care decisions.
- Educate families on health issues.

Implementation of a cross-culture education program enhances providers' awareness of how culture and social factors influence health care; helps providers understand how to interact with patients who have differing cultural viewpoints; and helps providers talk to and interact with these patients in a more effective way. The Office of Minority Health has published 14 national standards for health care organizations addressing culturally and linguistically appropriate services (CLAS) based on review of key laws, regulations, contracts, and standards currently used by federal and state agencies. A final report entitled "Assuring Cultural Competence in Health Care: Recommendations for National Standards and an Outcomes Focused Research Agenda" is available at www.omhrc.gov/CLAS [14]. Organizations that sponsor SBHCs may be familiar with CLAS and could be a resource in assisting school health center staff in developing culturally competent services. Possible resources could include interpreter services, educational materials, or staff to provide training on health practices of a particular cultural group. In addition, the American Medical Association has developed a workbook designed to provide practical information that can be used to enhance communication with adolescent patients. This guide offers suggestions for delivering individualized health care based on respect for and sensitivity to the multiple factors that define culture. *Delivering Culturally Effective Health Care to Adolescents* contains helpful background information, self-assessment, and additional resources and is available at www.ama-assn.org/ama1/pub/upload/mm/39/culturallyeffective.pdf [20].

Operational tools

Tools that are helpful in establishing and maintaining standards of care are critical to ensure that all clients receive the same quality of care. These tools serve as an integral part of an SBHC's Continuous Quality Improvement program. Policies and protocols that articulate the standards of care are an important mechanism to ensure quality services and to protect against inadvertent provider bias referred to earlier. All staff, not only direct service providers, should be included in the development of these policies and protocols and should be part of orientation for all new staff. A policy that states the specifics of the medical record review can help to ensure that clients are receiving the same standard of care regardless of race, ethnicity, or other factors. The medical record review policy should address the following elements: who reviews the records, how often the records are reviewed, and what processes exist to integrate information that requires further action. Peer review can be of particular benefit as it can prompt discussion among providers regarding best practice in specific areas. Satisfaction surveys can be an effective way to measure the individual client's satisfaction with the service provided. Information that evaluates the quality of cultural sensitivity can be determined by including questions such as, "did the provider you saw today understand why you came to the health center?" or "if English is not your first language, how easy was it to talk to the provider and did you understand the advice you were given?" It is important to incorporate information collected from the survey into one's practice. For instance, if language is identified to be a barrier to service, one must look at strategies to provide more linguistically appropriate services. These strategies may include using interpreter services, using patient education materials available in different languages, or recruiting staff who speak the language.

Client education

Some evidence exists that patient education efforts can make a difference in providing a higher level of culturally competent care. When a patient is able to ask questions and receive clear answers, that patient can participate more fully in the decision-making process [21]. Therefore, one way to increase patients' understanding of the services provided is to make books, pamphlets, or Internet sites available for school health center clients and their parents. These resources can prepare clients and families for what to expect during health encounters and specific examinations/procedure, and provide information about how to improve communication with the provider.

STUDENTS IN HEALTH CAREERS

The diverse students served in SBHCs are prime candidates to expose to opportunities for entry and training/education in health careers, especially high school students. Not only are these young people the workforce of the future, but many are motivated to plan for a job or field of study after graduation. In addition, many of these students speak two or more languages. What better way to increase the cultural diversity of the health care workforce than encouraging these youth to pursue a career in the field of health care? Students should recognize that competency in their primary language, if not English, is a valuable job skill. It is crucial for students to study their primary language and become competent in the verbal and written domains of that language. The ability to translate effectively could be used as a stepping stone to earn income while pursuing postsecondary studies, or as an integral part of their future careers.

One school-based health center's experience

There are many different ways to expose students to educational and employment opportunities in health careers. These methods can range from small initiatives using limited resources to a fully funded comprehensive program. This section discusses the experience of an SBHC in Chicago in developing their Students in Health Careers program. The SBHC is located in a typical medium-sized urban public high school. One of the unique characteristics of the school is its location in a community known as the port of entry for new immigrants to Chicago. The school boasts that it is one of the most diverse schools in the country, with students coming from over 60 countries and speaking more than 30 languages [22]. The SBHC's sponsoring agency is a not-for-profit community hospital that has been instrumental in assisting staff at the SBHC by providing resources to promote cultural competence. One example is the publication of *Cultural Spotlights,* a booklet highlighting the unique aspects of 13 different cultures, four religions, and the cultural aspects of pain [23]. The Students in Health Careers program uses three main strategies: a Health Careers Club, a collaborative relationship with the hospital to provide opportunities for students in health careers, and a scholarship program.

Health Careers Club

The Commission to End Heath Care Disparities suggests that increasing the entry of racial/ethnic minorities into health professional schools is one strategy to improve the delivery of culturally competent care [13]. The SBHC sponsors a club to promote entry into health careers. Recruitment of students includes working with school faculty and guidance counselors to identify students interested in health careers, and active recruitment by all health center staff in their individual contacts with students. Several speakers present at monthly meetings about topics chosen by the students. Some examples of speakers are staff from various disciplines in the hospital who highlight their professions; faculty from area community colleges who discuss specific program requirements and financial aid opportunities; and human resource staff from the hospital who discuss how to write a resume, apply for a job, and interview for a position.

One resource found to be of benefit is The Metropolitan Chicago Health Care Council's *Health Careers Guide* [24]. The guide includes information on specific careers, financial aid, schools, admissions testing, and a timeline for high school students. Although the target population for this guide is Illinois, much of the information can be helpful in other states. The guide is available at www.mchc.org/hcg [24].

Another resource found to be helpful is the Bureau of Health Professions' *Kids into Health Careers,* available at www.hrsa.gov/bhpr/kidscareers [25]. This national initiative was developed to supplement the pool of qualified applicants from economically and educationally disadvantaged and underrepresented minority populations for entry into health professions. An information packet is available online and includes examples of presentations to students, parents, and faculty. It also includes references for health professions, financial information, and federally funded health facilities.

Collaboration with the hospital

The school, hospital, and SBHC work collaboratively to provide opportunities for students to experience various health fields. The most successful events to date have included a Career Day at the school and a Health Career Day at the hospital. Each fall, the school sponsors a Career Day during which individuals from diverse professions present information about their jobs. Staff from the SBHC and hospital lead workshops for students who are interested in health careers. The most popular health careers identified by students are medicine and nursing, but other health careers are also included. Information about job requirements, job responsibilities, and salary range are presented. This type of live forum allows students to interact with various health professionals, ask questions, and determine more realistic expectations for creating a career path.

In the spring of the school year, the hospital sponsors a Health Careers Day at the hospital. Students are recruited from the Health Careers Club and other groups in the school that work with students to promote jobs after graduation. A small workgroup of representatives from the school, SBHC, and hospital plan the event. The day begins in the auditorium with an overview of hospital services and opportunities for students such as volunteering and performing community service projects. To expose students to multiple opportunities within the hospital system, the group is divided into three tracks. This division provides the opportunity for students to learn about entry-level positions in case they need a job after graduation to pay for their education. The tracks are as follows:

- The clinical track includes medicine, nursing, pharmacy, laboratory, radiology, and therapies (speech, occupational, and physical).
- The business track includes marketing, human resources, information systems, access services (admitting, scheduling, and registration), credit services (customer service, financial counseling, and collections), medical records, and child care.
- The service track includes housekeeping, engineering, security, storeroom, receiving, food service, and central service.

Students are divided into small groups and taken on an employee-led tour of the hospital. Numerous opportunities are available for students to interact with the tour guide and hospital staff. Evaluations from students and employees have been very positive and show great enthusiasm for the experience.

Less successful was the establishment of a mentoring program with students and hospital employees. Although a mentoring program can be a valuable strategy to provide students with hands-on experience, SBHC staff lacked the time and resources to devote to the program. However, for SBHCs interested in developing a mentoring or job shadowing program, a valuable resource is the Groundhog Job Shadow Initiative [26]. This national program is dedicated to engaging students in the world of work. Although the initiative is not specific to health careers, it does include helpful information and is available at www.jobshadow.org [26].

Health career scholarships

During the past few years, the SBHC has successfully raised funds to create scholarship awards for students interested in pursuing a health career. The ability to offer scholarships to students is a valuable tool as it provides an incentive for a student to begin the journey toward a specific health career. Students have typically used the scholarship to attend a Certified Nursing Assistant program so a part-time job could be held while preparing for entry into a nursing program or pursuing a nursing degree. A few students successfully enrolled in a university nursing program. The local chamber of commerce and medical staff at the sponsoring hospital have contributed donations to the scholarship fund. In the future, the school health center plans to approach more businesses in the community for donations to the scholarship fund. In addition, funding for a more comprehensive program in this area that would include mentoring and tutoring support for students interested in health careers will be sought.

SUMMARY

Attaining cultural competency in SBHCs is an evolving process that requires program staff to build the knowledge base and develop the skill level necessary to become culturally competent in service delivery. Most importantly, individual providers must have the desire to want to become culturally competent. Staff need to increase awareness of personal biases, as many are unaware of these biases and how they may impact the care provided. In addition, the students served by SBHCs are prime candidates to reach out to and enlist as future health professionals, as many of these students possess the capacity and interest for such a career and are also bilingual and bicultural. These students of the present can increase the cultural diversity and improve the cultural competency of the health care workforce of the future.

Acknowledgments

The author would like to acknowledge the staff at The Health Center at Roosevelt High School and Swedish Covenant Hospital in Chicago, Ill, for their tremendous commitment to the students, and Beth Blacksin, MS, RN, for assistance in editing this manuscript.

References

[1] National Assembly on School-Based Health Care. School-based health centers: a child-focused safety net strategy. Available at: www.nasbhc.org. Accessed February 14, 2005.

[2] Cross T, Bazron B, Dennis K, et al. Towards a Culturally competent system of care: a monograph of effective services for minority children who are severely emotionally disturbed, vol. 1. Washington (DC): CASSP Technical Assistance Center, Georgetown University Child Care Development Training Center; 1989.

[3] Rodriguez J, Cauce A, Wilson L. A Conceptual framework of identity formation in a society of multiple cultures. Seattle (WA): The Casey Family Programs; 2000.

[4] National Assembly on School-Based Health Care. School-based health centers national census school year 2001–2002. Available at: www.nasbhc.org/EQ/2001census/characteristics.pdf. Accessed November 14, 2004.

[5] Census Bureau. Projections of the total resident population by 5-year age groups, race, and Hispanic origin with special age categories: middle series, 1999–2000. Available at: www.census.gov/population/projections/nation/summary/np-t4-b.txt. Accessed November 16, 2004.

[6] Census Bureau. Projections of the total resident population by 5-year age groups, race, and Hispanic origin with special age categories: middle series, 2011–2015. Available at: www.census.gov/population/projections/nation/summary/np-t4-d.txt. Accessed November 16, 2004.

[7] The Center for Health and Health Care in Schools. This land was made for you and me: cultural competence in school-based health centers, January 2004. Available at: www.healthinschools.org/sh/cultpaper.abs. Accessed November 16, 2004.

[8] US Department of Health and Human Services. Protecting the health of minority communities. HHS Disparities initiative: Fact Sheet. Available at: www.omhrc.gov/rah/index-new.htm. Accessed February 7, 2005.

[9] Wasserman RC, Croft CA, Brotherton SE. Preschool vision screening in a pediatric practice: a study from the Pediatric Research on Office Settings (PROS) Network. Pediatrics 1992;89: 834–8.

[10] Hahn BA. Children's health: racial and ethnic differences in the use of prescriptive medications. Pediatrics 1995;95:727–32.

[11] Finkelstein JA, Brown RA, Schneider LC, et al. Quality of care for preschool children with asthma: the role of social factors and practice setting. Pediatrics 1995;95:389–94.

[12] Institute of Medicine. Unequal treatment: what healthcare providers need to know about racial and ethnic disparities in healthcare. 2002. Available at: www.iom.edu/Object. File/Master/4/175/0.pdf. Accessed February 7, 2005.

[13] The Center for Health and Health Care in Schools. New commission to end health disparities in health care, volume 5, number 12, February 2005. Available at: www.healthinschools. org/ejournal/2005.feb1.html. Accessed February 7, 2005.

[14] US Department of Health and Human Services. Health Resources and Services Administration, Office of Minority Health, national standards for culturally and linguistically appropriate services in health care: final report. Washington, DC, March 2001. Available at: www.omhrc.gov/clas/index.htm. Accessed January 11, 2005.

[15] National Association of School Psychologists, The Provision of Culturally Competent Services in the School Setting, Fact Sheet. Available at: www.nasponline.org/cultural competence/provision cultcompsvcs.html. Accessed November 11, 2004.

[16] Campinha-Bacote J. The process of cultural competence in the delivery of healthcare services: a model of care. Journal of Transcultural Nursing 2002;13(3):181–4.

[17] US Department of Health and Human Services, Health Resources and Services Administration. Definitions of cultural competence. Reviewed 2002. Available at: www.bhpr.hrsa. gov/diversity/cultcomp.htm. Accessed November 11, 2004.

[18] Flores G, Abreu M, Scwartz I, et al. The Importance of language and culture in pediatric care: case studies from the Latino community. J Pediatr 2000;137(6):842–8.

[19] Flores G. Culture and the patient-physician relationship: achieving cultural competency in health care. J Pediatr 2000;136:14–23.

[20] American Medical Association. Delivering culturally effective health care to adolescents. Available at: www.ama.org/ama1/pub/upload/mm/39/culturallyeffective.pdf. Accessed January 11, 2005.

[21] Institute of Medicine, What healthcare consumers need to know about racial and ethnic disparities in healthcare. March 2002. Available at: www.iom.edu/Object.File/Master/ 4/176/0.pdf. Accessed February 7, 2005.

[22] Roosevelt High School. Profile 2003–04. Available at: www.Roosevelt.cps.k12.il.us. Accessed February 14, 2005.

[23] Swedish Covenant Hospital. Cultural spotlights. Chicago (IL): Swedish Convent Hospital; 2002.

[24] Metropolitan Chicago Healthcare Council. Health careers guide, 2004. Available at: www.mchc.org/hcg. Accessed February 27, 2004.

[25] US Department of Health and Human Services. Health Resources and Services Administration, kids into health careers. Available at: www.hrsa.gov/bhpr/kidscareers. Accessed February 27, 2004.

[26] Job Shadowing. How to have a successful groundhog job shadow day. Available at: www.jobshadow.org. Accessed February 27, 2004.

Nurs Clin N Am 40 (2005) 649–660

NURSING CLINICS
OF NORTH AMERICA

ELSEVIER
SAUNDERS

Beyond the Physical Examination: the Nurse Practitioner's Role in Adolescent Risk Reduction and Resiliency Building in a School-Based Health Center

Teresa K. Davis, APN, MSN, WHNP

Loyola University Chicago, Niehoff School of Nursing, 6525 North Sheridan Road, Chicago, IL 60626, USA

School-based health centers (SBHCs) in high schools provide a unique setting in which to deliver risk-reduction and resilience-building services to adolescents. The traditional health care system operating in the United States focuses on the treatment of illness and disease rather than on preventing problems originating from health risk behaviors [1]. Nurse practitioners can promote healthy behavior in adolescents through linkages to parents, schools, and community organizations; by conducting individual risk assessments; and by providing health education and access to creative health programs that build resilience and promote protective factors. With a focus on wellness, nurse practitioners as advanced practice nurses and specialists in disease prevention and health promotion can establish students' health priorities in the context of the primary health care they deliver on a daily basis.

DEVELOPMENTAL STAGES AND RISK BEHAVIORS

Navigating the transition from childhood to adulthood is difficult for many adolescents. Psychologist Eric Erikson [2] described "identity versus role confusion" as the ability to form an identity and achieve adult autonomy. This is the developmental task of adolescence. More recently, adolescent development has been divided into three stages: early adolescence is 11 to 14 years of age or junior high aged; middle adolescence is 15 to 17 years of age or high school aged; and late adolescence is 18 to 21 years of age or college/work aged [3]. Each stage is characterized by different behaviors and variable cognitive, physical, social, and emotional developmental changes [3]. An awareness of these stages and changes by health care providers is important to support adolescents as they mature into adulthood.

The leading causes of mortality in the adolescent age group are motor vehicle crashes and other unintentional injuries; homicide; and suicide [1]. These

E-mail address: tkaydavis@msn.com

0029-6465/05/$ – see front matter
doi:10.1016/j.cnur.2005.07.010

deaths are the result of preventable risk factors. The Youth Risk Behavior Surveillance survey documents that many high school students engage in behaviors that increase their chance of death: 44.9% use alcohol; 30.2% have ridden with a drunk driver; and 17.1% carried a weapon in the 30 days preceding the survey [1]. Engaging in risky behaviors can lead to adverse health outcomes and these behaviors can affect adolescents' current and future health status [4]. It is important for nurse practitioners and other health professionals working with adolescents to become aware of and address these serious risk factors.

HEALTHY PEOPLE 2010—CRITICAL HEALTH OBJECTIVES FOR ADOLESCENTS

Risk factors that affect the health and well-being of adolescents may be conceptualized within the framework of Healthy People 2010. Behaviors such as tobacco use; unhealthy dietary habits; inadequate physical activity; alcohol and other drug use; and behaviors that result in violence and unintentional injuries are targeted as critical objectives to improve the health of adolescents [1].

Risk behaviors and conditions may be categorized into various groups. These groups include medical conditions (eg, chronic and acute illnesses); nutrition issues (eg, obesity, eating disorders, poor eating habits); mental health problems (eg, depression, hopelessness, suicidal ideation); psychosocial factors (eg, chaotic home life, poverty, violence, problems with peers); safety (eg, unintentional injury, lack of seat belt use, homicide, sports injuries); sexual/reproductive problems (eg, pregnancy, sexually transmitted disease [STD], HIV/AIDS); and substance abuse and tobacco use. These risk behaviors reflect the risks outlined in the "21 Critical Health Objectives" for adolescents summarized in Healthy People 2010. However, any categorization of risk behaviors fails to take into account that all these factors are interrelated. Thus, a comprehensive approach to risk reduction, which includes interventions at the individual, family, school, and community level, is likely to be most effective.

Adolescent health research suggests that identified health risks may be reduced through building resiliency [4–6]. According to researchers, parent–family relationships, school connectedness, a sense of future, high self-esteem, community involvement, an interested adult, and academic success are protective factors found in resilient individuals that help reduce health risks [5,7]. Thus, interventions to promote resiliency must address the whole person within the context of school, family, and community.

COMPREHENSIVE RISK ASSESSMENT

A comprehensive risk assessment is the first step in identifying the health status of adolescents. Nurse practitioners, mental health professionals, health educators, registered nurses, and social workers should conduct a comprehensive risk assessment of each student presenting for care, using a formal screening tool or through a comprehensive verbal history from the student.

The Guideline for Adolescent Preventive Services (GAPS) self-report questionnaire is the "gold standard" for risk assessment [8]. It was developed by the American Medical Association in 1994 to address adolescent preventive services in outpatient clinical settings. The GAPS tool includes a risk assessment questionnaire, recommendations for health screenings, and anticipatory guidance strategies. The GAPS Initial Adolescent Questionnaire is a four-page survey designed for adolescents to complete individually. The questionnaire may require 30 to 60 minutes for a student to complete. Once completed, the forms should be reviewed with the student to identify behavioral risk areas or areas in which the student requests additional information. A shorter self-reported Student Health Survey (Fig. 1), or a comprehensive history and physical form that includes risk assessment questions (the "Initial Adolescent Visit") (Fig. 2), may be used if there are time constraints during the initial visit. However, the GAPS questionnaire should be administered during a subsequent visit by the nurse practitioner, physician, psychologist, social worker, registered nurse, or health educator. If another health care provider conducts the GAPS assessment, the nurse practitioner should review it to continue risk reduction strategies in follow-up visits. In addition to GAPS, there are other preventive health programs, including Bright Futures [9] and Put Prevention Into Practice [10]. A combination of these programs may be necessary to meet the individual needs of students.

At the initial SBHC visit, the comprehensive services provided by the SBHC and the patient confidentiality policy should be explained before beginning the history or risk assessment. Most young people present with several risk factors. The primary care provider should determine what issues are impacting the student's current health status and prioritize them to begin risk reduction interventions. A typical assessment may uncover an adolescent who is overweight; drinks occasionally; is sexually active and at risk for an STD; and who has limited support at home. However, this same student may have close ties to the school, be on a school sports team, and have a close relationship with the coach. Another student might express depressed feelings or suicide ideation, which must be addressed and assessed immediately to determine if intervention and referral to a mental health professional is necessary. If the student is having passive thoughts of death and feelings of helplessness but no true suicide ideation, then a plan needs to be developed. The student would benefit from psychological counseling and a safety contract between the student and the health care provider.

Risk factors should be noted in a systematic way on the student's medical record. Using a "Problem List" or creating a flow sheet that is placed in the front of the student's chart prompts health care providers to address ongoing risk factors and promote continuity of care during follow-up visits.

A nurse practitioner can feel overwhelmed when an adolescent presents with multiple risk behaviors during an appointment for a simple sport's physical. The student may not understand why the nurse practitioner is asking in-depth and personal questions about sex or drug use when the student just wants

STUDENT HEALTH SURVEY

We would like you to answer these questions while you wait. We will go over your answers with you and may talk to you about areas that could affect your health. *Your answers will not be shared with anyone outside the school based health center.* You do not have to answer any questions you don't want to. If you have any questions or health problems please feel free to discuss them with us. *Answers are completely confidential.*

Name:_____   Grade:_____   Date:_____

ID#_____   Gender: □ Male □ Female   Age:_____

1. Do you eat breakfast everyday   □ No   □ Yes

2. How many servings of fruits and vegetables do you eat a day? (circle one)
   A. 0-1   B. 2-3   C. 4-5   D. 5+

3. Are you doing well in school?   □ No   □ Yes

4. Have you been in a fight or suspended from school in the last year?   □ Yes   □ No

5. What do you plan to do when you finish high school? (circle one)
   A. college   B. military   C. voc/tech school
   D. work   E. don't know   F. other_____

6. Have you tried to lose weight during the past year?   □ Yes   □ No

7. Do you currently exercise or participate in activities that get your whole body moving (walking, jogging, bicycling, dancing, etc.) for at least 30 minutes at a time, at least 5 days a week?   □ No   □ Yes

8. Do you smoke cigarettes/cigars, use snuff or chew tobacco?   □ Yes   □ No

9. Do you use marijuana or other drugs, or inhalants?   □ Yes   □ No

10. Do you always wear a seat belt when you're in a car?   □ No   □ Yes

11. Do you drink alcohol?   □ Yes   □ No

12. Do you ever drive after drinking or when you are high?   □ Yes   □ No

13. Do you use a helmet when riding a bike, rollerblading or skateboarding?   □ No   □ Yes

14. Do you ever get into a car when the driver has been drinking or is high?   □ Yes   □ No

15. Do you think you are or could be gay/lesbian/ homosexual/bisexual?   □ Yes   □ No

16. Have you ever had sexual intercourse?   (By sexual intercourse we mean vaginal, oral, or anal)   □Yes   □No

17. Are you doing something to prevent yourself from getting Sexually Transmitted Diseases (STDs), HIV/AIDS?   □Yes (circle one or more)   □ No
   A.*not having sex*
   B. using condoms every time
   C. *other*_____

18. Have you ever been physically, sexually, or verbally threatened or abused?   □Yes   □No

19. Are you worried about violence or your safety at home or school?   □ Yes   □ No

20. Are you teased or picked on?   □Yes   □No

21. In the past month, have you often felt sad or depressed?   □Yes   □No

22. Do you have someone you feel you can talk to?   □No   □Yes

23. Is there an adult in your life that you can count on, other than School Based Health Center staff?   □No   □Yes

24. Have you ever thought about, planned or tried to kill or hurt yourself?   □Yes   □No

25. Do you carry a gun or a weapon to school?   □Yes   □No

26. Are there any guns, hunting rifles or weapons in your home?   □Yes   □No

27. Is there any thing else you would like to talk about today?   _____

Staff:

Date:

Fig. 1. Student health survey.

a sports physical. Primary care providers must be proactive in explaining that the SBHC provides comprehensive care, and that the staff is concerned about the overall health of students and not just the reason for the visit on that particular day.

During their visits, it is recommended that students be educated on health risks identified in their questionnaire and given resource materials, such as

<u>INITIAL **Adolescent Visit**</u>   (page 1 of 2)

Date:_____   **Name:**

Reason for visit: _____

_____

Past Medical History   *PCP:* _____ *Ins?*_____

Meds: _____ Allergies: _____
Surgery: _____ Hospitalizations: _____
Transfusion: _____ Chronic Illness/birth defect: _____
Childhood diseases: *chicken pox?*_____Other_____
Immunizations: _____TB test: _____Last eye exam:_____Vision Prob?_____
Last Dental Exam: _____ *Brushing habits:*_____ *Flossing:* _____

Family History

Mother-alive & well or _____ Father-alive & well or _____
Stroke _____ Cancer _____ Heart disease _____ Hypertension _____ Diabetes _____
Liver dis. _____ Sickle cell _____ Genetic _____ Psychiatric _____
Substance Abuse _____ Other _____

Social History

Grade _____ Level of Achievement (honor roll/probation) _____
Sports/After school activities _____ Living arrangements _____
D.V./Sex. Abuse _____ Counseling _____ Coping Strategies _____
Depression/S.I./Attempts _____Anger/Violence_____
Safety: weapons, seat belts, helmets, fights_ _____
__Tobacco _____ Partner/family _____
__Alcohol _____ Partner/family _____Drive under influence?_____
__Drugs _____Partner/family _____
Nutrition _____Eating disorder _____Caffeine_____ Exercise _____
Future Plans _____Spirituality _____ Strengths/Assets _____

Sexual History

Ever had sex? ____yes ____no Age first coitus _____   #lifetime partners _____ Current Partner __yes __no
                                                                          #partners last 30 days: _____
Type: (circle) O   A   V   Other _____
History STD _____ Partner w/risk behaviors _____

Females: Menarche _____ LMP _____ Length _____ Interval _____ Flow _____
Gravida ____ Para_____ Pregnancy History: _____
Menstrual problems _____ Previous Pap/pelvic _____ Abn pap _____
Gyne problems _____ Previous contraceptive use _____
Contraception preference _____ Planning pregnancy within next year? _____

Males: Ever fathered a child _____ Condom use: _____
Genital warts/lesions/discharge _____ Other: _____

Review of Systems

HEENT _____ Chest/lungs _____ Palpitations _____
Exercise intolerance _____ Breast problems _____SBE?_____Abd. Pain _____
N/V/D _____ Bowel _____ Pelvic pain _____ Dysuria _____
Scrotal pain/testicular pain _____STE?_____Vaginal/penile discharge _____
Testicular lump _____ Genital lesions _____ Rectal pain/lesions _____
Back pain _____ Extremity pain/swelling _____ Skin rash/lesion _____
Sleep problems _____ Any questions about body?_____ *(Continued Next Page)*

Fig. 2. Initial adolescent visit.

PROVIDER SIGNATURE:

(Continued from previous page) ***Date:*** _____   ***Page 2 of 2***   ***Name:***

Physical Exam

Ht _____   Wt _____   B/P _____   P _____   R_____

BMI: _____   Temp_____

	Nml	Abn	Comments
General			
Skin			
Head			
Ears			
Eyes			
Nose			
Throat/Mouth			
Thyroid			
Neck			
Lungs			
Heart			
Breasts			
Breasts/Tanner			
Abdomen			
Pubic Hair/Tanner			
Groin (M)/Vulva (F)			
Penis/Vagina			
Scrotum/Cervix			
Testes/Uterus			
Adnexae			
Anus/Rectum			
Extremities			
Spine			
Neuro			

Assessment:

_____

_____

_____

_____

_____

Plan:

_____

_____

_____

_____

_____

RTC: _____   **Brochures/Supplies/Referrals:**_____

Provider Signature: _____

Fig. 2 (continued)

brochures, pamphlets, and books such as *Healthy Life: Student's Self-Care Guide*, that address health risk factors, problems, and education topics specific to adolescents [11]. These interventions help reinforce the topics covered during the initial visit. Once risk status has been determined, the nurse practitioner or another multidisciplinary team member can formulate a plan with the student for risk reduction. This plan may include individual approaches such as screening, treatment, and health education, or group approaches such as encouraging students to join activities like life skills or weight loss groups. A combination of individual and group approaches that help to reduce risk by building resiliency and protective factors is likely to be most effective.

CONFIDENTIALITY—THE NEED TO SHARE INFORMATION

In an SBHC setting, it is extremely important for adolescents to know their confidentiality rights and limits to confidentiality when engaging with SBHC staff. A trusting, confidential relationship must be in place between health care providers and students to obtain an accurate and honest risk assessment. Nurse practitioners and other health care providers are responsible for knowing federal and state regulations on consent laws. These laws and regulations vary from state to state. Adolescents should be informed as to which services and treatments are available to them at the SBHC without their parent's permission, and which information/treatment provided must by state law be shared with their parents. Students need to understand that personal information is not shared with others except in life-threatening cases or if a student is a danger to himself or others.

There are several different mechanisms to make students understand patient confidentiality. It is important to have a clear policy delineating SBHC personnel's responsibilities for maintaining a confidential environment. The office manger or receptionist may be delegated to explain the SBHC's confidentiality policy to a student when they first register for an appointment. They may also be responsible for the student signing the confidentiality statement, which becomes part of the health record and acknowledges that the student has read and understands the agreement. The confidentiality statement should be posted in the waiting room and every examination/counseling room. Each clinician should talk to the students about the confidentiality policy, ensuring that the adolescent is aware of the nature of their relationship before the provider begins to ask probing and personal questions during a risk assessment. Students must have assurance of confidentiality to provide an honest accounting of behavioral risks. Maintaining a high level of trust and security must be a priority among all the staff members of an SBHC.

Adolescents must also be made aware of the difference between high school staff and SBHC staff. This practice is because state and federal laws on health data confidentiality may differ from state and federal laws on privacy of education information. Nurse practitioners operate within the contractual agreement the SBHC has with the host school. These agreements, however, often place limitations on providing comprehensive care. For example, many SBHCs do not dispense contraceptives to students because of school administration concerns over community values. All staff must be aware of and follow protocols established by the SBHCs for referrals to outside agencies for family planning health care services.

TRUST AND AUTHENTICITY

Nurse practitioners are educated to understand that building trust is the single most important factor when treating and caring for adolescents. Students are more likely to respond positively when they feel that a health care professional is authentic. Active listening; setting goals with the student with clear plans for follow-up; referring the adolescent to programs that are meaningful and meet individual needs; responding to individual differences; and creating access for drop-in visits when a student just needs to talk are all positive ways to reinforce and enhance authenticity in the relationship.

Remembering the unique characteristics of each student and recalling the student's health problems or risk factors are ideal. However, in a large and busy clinical setting it is often difficult to remember every student. Making specific and detailed notes on the initial health record about the student's family and social situation and about resiliency factors, such as future goals and dreams, is one way to remember. These notes can help health care providers respond in a genuine, meaningful, and caring manner. A specially designed initial history and physical form works well for this documentation and functions as a risk assessment tool if the student hasn't yet completed a formal self-report risk assessment such as the GAPS.

There are many different ways to establish rapport and place the student at ease. One way is to begin the conversation with a statement such as,

> "I work for you. My job is to find out your strengths and identify what factors are affecting your health in a negative way. I want to uncover any health problems you might have and work with you to help you stay healthy and be successful in school and in life. I need your help to find things that may be affecting your health now or in the future; that's why I'd like to ask you some personal questions. Once we do our detective work together, then we can discuss any factors that may affect your health. The goal is to work together so that you leave high school as an expert on your own health. I do not share your personal information with anyone without asking your permission, except in certain cases which you just read about in the patient confidentiality section on the registration form."

The message must be clear that achieving good health is a collaborative and ongoing effort between a health care provider and the student. Students respond when they feel that confidential information is protected and that they are part of the plan. Students appreciate having their voice heard and feeling respected.

PROGRAMS FOR BUILDING RESILIENCE AND PROTECTIVE FACTORS

A needs assessment to determine the most prevalent risk behaviors among adolescents in a school should be conducted before health promotion programs are developed. Health record reviews may help determine population health risk trends. For example, periodic health record/reviews can help to determine the prevalence of obesity, sexual activity, unintended pregnancy, STD, tobacco/alcohol/drug use, depression/suicide, and risks to safety among the SBHC population. SBHC staff should prioritize their efforts by addressing the most prevalent problems in their adolescent population. Programs and activities can then be developed to address these risk factors and reinforce protective factors.

Data from the National Longitudinal Study on Adolescent Health identified parent–family connectedness and perceived school connectedness as powerful protective factors for students [6]. Other protective factors include sense of future, high self-esteem, an interested adult, academic success, and community involvement [3]. The SBHC team can use this information to develop risk reduction strategies and build resiliency for students in their care.

SBHCs are uniquely situated to provide a "home base" for adolescents, connecting them to health information, school activities, and school friends. Providing a student-friendly environment allows students to spend their lunch hour or other free time visiting the SBHC, further connecting them to staff that they trust and respect and who serve as positive role models. The SBHC staff help bolster students' self-esteem and a sense of future while filling the role of an interested adult for adolescents.

It is important that SBHCs develop specific programs to foster resilience-building skills and increase the protective factor of school connectedness. Input from the student population is important when developing programs and activities. It is also essential to consider the availability of qualified staff. Some SBHCs have a health educator whose responsibility it is to create and deliver programs. SBHCs without a health educator could rely on other health professionals to design programs that address the needs of students. Community partners can also be recruited to deliver programs in the school and community.

RESILIENCY-BUILDING PROGRAMS

Creating and implementing resiliency programs is a team effort. Our SBHC is sponsored by Loyola University Chicago and is directed by a School of Nursing faculty member. We are fortunate to have a team consisting of a nurse practitioner, family practice physician, clinical psychologist, health educator, and medical assistant/receptionist. The SBHC serves as a site for undergraduate and graduate nursing students and dietetic, psychology, and medical students, and is funded by federal Health Resources Services Administration grants, state of Illinois funds, and numerous private foundations. The programs described below reflect the needs of students and the talents and creativity of SBHC staff.

The Nutrition Revolution

The Nutrition Revolution is a comprehensive nutrition program developed to address poor nutritional habits and significant overweight/obesity rates in an adolescent population. The Nutrition Revolution involves making the SBHC a "Junk Free Zone" where students are asked to trade their junk food for a healthy snack or to put away the junk food while they are visiting the SBHC. Students are also provided healthy snacks if they miss lunch because of an SBHC appointment or if they work after school on SBHC projects. If students are overweight or obese, referrals are made to the nurse practitioner or to dietetic students who intern at the SBHC. Students meet one-on-one with the nurse practitioner or dietetic intern. An individual weight loss plan is developed for them in addition to nutritional counseling, exercise, and assistance with planning daily meals. The SBHC takes a stand for healthy eating and students perceive the importance that adult role models place on taking care of one's body. Feeling good about oneself is an important component of resiliency.

Cooking with Heart and Soul

Cooking with Heart and Soul is a nutrition education program designed to enhance family and school connectedness—important resiliency factors. High school students and their families, including siblings, meet evenings once a week for 6 weeks and learn to cook nutritious and delicious meals with the help of guest chefs such as school administrators, the school's security guard, parents, School of Nursing faculty, family of SBHC personnel, and various other volunteers. SBHC staff, guest chefs, and dietetic interns work with families to prepare the meals and clean up afterwards. Participants receive educational tips on healthy eating and exercise and are given information on stress reduction, teen–parent communication, and coping skills. Topics such as "Good Choices if You Must Eat Fast Food," "Stress and Eating," and "Comfort Foods—Why Do We Crave Them?" elicit discussions among participants. Cooking with Heart and Soul allows family members to share the happenings of their day with one another, helps neighbors to know neighbors, and helps parents to know their children better. Programming of this nature does require additional external funding and support of staff and administration. Donations of food from local grocery chains help sustain the program.

Future Health Professionals

Future Health Professionals is a club that was developed by the SBHC's nurse practitioner for at-risk adolescents who are unsure of their future and want to learn more about health and allied health careers. The health careers club can help students see the relationship between academic performance and their future endeavors. Students learn about various health careers and health care topics from guest speakers such as nursing and medical students and health professionals from the university academic health center. Activities offered by the club include college preparation sessions, cardiopulmonary resuscitation certification, field trips to health career colleges, and health-related demonstrations such as proper hand washing. Adolescents who attend the Future Health Professionals group feel more connected to SBHC staff and each other and feel comfortable speaking to staff about their future career options, which are important resiliency factors.

Teen Talk and Living 101

Teen Talk and Living 101 are forums for adolescents to discuss mental health issues that are important to them. The SBHC psychologist developed these programs to promote mental health awareness and teach students life skills and healthy coping strategies. Discussions and role playing on how to resolve conflicts with peers, for example, give students the tools to protect and prepare them for real-life situations. The social and emotional well-being of adolescents is enhanced through these discussions. Students' mental health supports and protective factors are also strengthened. The groups are offered during the students' lunch period or after school. The SBHC provides a confidential meeting place for participants, and healthy snacks.

Healthy Teens

Healthy Teens is an advocacy program that trains high school students to be role models and peer educators for grammar school youth in their community. Teen advocates are trained in teamwork and advocacy skills and work with grammar school students to foster social skills and improve self-image. These are important resiliency factors for grammar school youth. Community leaders, who have an interest in the health and welfare of youth, act as role models to the "Healthy Teens," providing them with a positive support system that may be lacking in their own homes. After-school and community-school initiatives such as Healthy Teens strengthen connectedness among students, teachers, families, and group leaders. Many "Healthy Teens" choose to become peer mentors in the high school. They provide individual and group sessions to their peers on topics such as sexually transmitted infection (STI) prevention, conflict resolution, and unintended pregnancies. Healthy Teens has been operating for over 10 years and is way for students to contribute to their school, peers, and community.

Walking Club

The Walking Club was developed to interest students in weight loss and exercise. The Walking Club meets after school, 3 to 4 days each week in the spring and fall months. Students, teachers, and SBHC staff walk for one half to three quarters of an hour with members of the SBHC team on the high school track field or in inclement weather in the school halls. Because walking facilitates conversation, students often share their concerns and problems with SBHC staff. The informal and less structured nature of walking helps students connect to positive role models and also improve their health and well-being. Exercise is an important component in managing one's weight, and a club that focuses and supports student exercise can improve adolescents' self-esteem and sense of worth, which are important resiliency factors.

In addition to these comprehensive programs created by SBHC staff, many schools provide after-school and in-school clubs for students. SBHC health care providers should become knowledgeable about school programs to establish a clear referral system. The SBHC can post flyers about school programs in the health center so that students can obtain information about upcoming events or meetings. Assisting students with referrals, giving written information, allowing adolescents to use the phone, and introducing them to the teacher or counselor involved in the school program help build resiliency by showing genuine interest in students' activities.

SUMMARY

Nurse practitioners in an SBHC provide access to creative health programs and conduct school and physical examinations and screenings for pregnancy, obesity, and STIs on a daily basis. As health promoters and disease prevention specialists, nurse practitioners in SBHCs should go beyond the physical examination to conduct risk assessments and develop activities to foster resiliency for adolescents. Establishing a trusting relationship is a key component to effective risk reduction. Health care providers have unique roles in SBHCs and can make a difference in students' health by assisting at-risk adolescents in becoming strong, sound, and healthy adults.

References

[1] Centers for Disease Control and Prevention, National Center for Chronic Disease Prevention and Health Promotion, Division of Adolescent and School Health. Health Resources and Services Administration, Maternal and Child Health Bureau, Office of Adolescent Health, National Adolescent Health Information Center, University of California, San Francisco. Improving the health of adolescents and young adults: a guide for states and communities. Atlanta (GA): Centers for Disease Control and Prevention; 2004.

[2] Erikson E. Childhood and society. New York: W.W. Norton; 1950.

[3] Dunn AM, Fischer JW. Developmental management of adolescents. In: Burns CE, Dunn MA, Brady MA, et al, editors. Pediatric primary care: a handbook for nurse practitioners. 3rd edition. St. Louis (MO): Saunders; 2004. p. 151–69.

[4] Rew L, Horner SD. Youth resilience framework for reducing health-risk behaviors in adolescents. J Pediatr Nurs 2003;18(6):379–88.

[5] Burt MR. Reasons to invest in adolescents. J Adolesc Health 2002;31(Suppl 6):S136–52.

[6] Resnick MD, Bearman PS, Blum RW, et al. Protecting adolescents from harm. Findings from the National Longitudinal Study on Adolescent Health. JAMA 1997;278(10):823–32.

[7] Lammers C, Ireland M, Resnick M, et al. Influences on adolescents' decision to postpone onset of sexual intercourse: a survival analysis of virginity among youths aged 13–18 years. J Adolesc Health 2000;26:42–8.

[8] Elster AB, Kuznets NJ. GAPS (Guidelines for Adolescent Preventive Services). Available at: http://ama-assn.org/ama/pub/category/1980.html. Accessed 1994.

[9] Bright Futures. Guidelines for health supervision and infants, children and adolescents, September 2002. Available at: http://brightfutures.aap.org.

[10] Agency for Healthcare Research and Quality. Put Prevention Into Practice. Available at: http://www.ahrq.gov/ppip/ppipabou.htm. Accessed May 2000.

[11] Powell DR. Healthy life: student's self-care guide. 2nd edition. American Institute for Preventive Medicine. Available at: www.HealthyLife.com. Accessed 2001.

Nurs Clin N Am 40 (2005) 661–669

NURSING CLINICS
OF NORTH AMERICA

ELSEVIER
SAUNDERS

Childhood Obesity: a School-Based Approach to Increase Nutritional Knowledge and Activity Levels

Beth Edwards, RN, MSN, BC, FNP

34980 Sarah Lane, Denham Springs, LA 70706, USA

OVERVIEW

O besity is a complex chronic condition caused by a lack of physical activity and increased caloric consumption. Approximately 300,000 people die each year from obesity-related conditions, making it one of this country's most significant illnesses. In the United States, only tobacco use causes more preventable deaths [1]. Healthy People 2010, a National initiative, has designated overweight and obesity as leading health indicators [2].

Although there are genetic factors and certain health conditions that contribute to obesity, it is predominately influenced by the environment [3]. A major environmental factor influencing the obesity rate is the lack of physical activity. Accepted societal behaviors, such as driving instead of walking or riding a bicycle, or using elevators rather than climbing stairs, contribute to sedentary lifestyles. More than 60% of adult and adolescent Americans are physically underactive [4]. Much of this underactivity can be attributed to the amount of time spent watching television and playing video games. It is estimated that adults spend an average of 2 hours per day watching television whereas children and adolescents spend an average of 25 hours per week doing the same. One out of every five children and adolescents watch television an average of 35 hours per week [5]. Other than sleeping, children spend more time watching television than any other activity. By the time they reach 18 years of age, the average teenager has spent more time watching television than learning in the classroom [5,6].

The consumption of readily available high calorie foods is another environmental factor influencing obesity rates. It is estimated that 60% of women are employed and spend fewer than 10 hours per week preparing meals [7]. More

This work was partially supported by a grant from the Baton Rouge Area Foundation and the Agency for Health Care Research and Quality (AHRQ) grant HS 11834.

E-mail address: Beth2430@aol.com

people are turning to food prepared by restaurants and fast food chains, taking full advantage of the ability to "super size" the portions. Typically, these meals are higher in fat, sodium, and calories than food prepared at home. It is estimated that approximately 46% of American adults eat out on any given day of the week [8].

Schools are required to follow USDA Dietary Guidelines for the school lunch program, but not for foods sold in snack bars, vending machines, and a la carte in the lunch line [2]. Many schools find it difficult to resist the incentives that vending machine operators and soft drink companies offer for allowing sugary sodas and junk food to be dispersed. Profits from these sales often support sports teams and after-school activities.

Obesity costs our health care system $117 billion per year in direct medical expenses. This figure does not include indirect expenses such as lost wages and decreased productivity. In his speech at the 2003 Innovation in Prevention Awards Gala, Tommy Thompson [9], the Secretary of the Department of Health and Human Services, stated, "The cost to US businesses of obesity-related health problems in 1994 added up to almost $13 billion, with $8 billion of this going toward health insurance expenditures, $2.4 billion for sick leave, $1.8 billion for life insurance and close to $1 billion for disability insurance."

PREVALENCE

According to the National Health and Nutrition Examination Survey, the prevalence of obesity in men and women aged 20 to 74 years increased from 13.4% in 1960 to 1962 to a staggering 30.9% in 1999 to 2000 [10]. This prevalence translates into an estimated 64% of adult Americans or 110 million people who are either overweight or obese [11]. These same individuals are at risk for hypertension, type 2 diabetes, heart disease, orthopedic problems, stroke, certain cancers, and depression [1].

Also of great concern are recent studies that report a dramatic increase in the prevalence of children who are overweight. Data from the National Longitudinal Survey of Youth (NLSY) has revealed an overweight prevalence of 21.5% among African American children, 21.8% among Hispanic children, and 12.3% among non-Hispanic Whites. These data represent a 120% increase in the prevalence of overweight among African American and Hispanic children and a 50% increase among non-Hispanic Whites from 1986 to 1998. The NLSY provides the most recent available data based on a single, high-quality, nationally representative sample [12].

SHORT- AND LONG-TERM CONSEQUENCES OF OVERWEIGHT AMONG SCHOOL-AGED CHILDREN

Childhood obesity has several short-term medical risks, including abnormal glucose tolerance, high cholesterol values, high blood pressure, and bone and joint disorders. Obese children are more than twice as likely to have high blood pressure or heart disease as children who are of normal weight [13].

Long-term consequences include depression, social discrimination, and increased behavioral problems. Obese children are often ridiculed and teased with subsequent exclusion from groups and activities. They often have low self-esteem and report increased rates of sadness and loneliness, and may be more likely to use alcohol and tobacco [14]. Children who are overweight have a significantly higher risk for becoming overweight adults, which in turn is associated with a higher prevalence of heart disease, type 2 diabetes, and cancer [15]. In 2001, Styne [16] reported that obese adolescents have an 8.5- to 10-fold risk for adulthood hypertension. In 1990, only 4% of childhood diabetes was diagnosed as type 2. Today that number ranges from 8% to 48% depending on age and ethnicity [17].

RATIONALE FOR THE PROGRAM

A literature search revealed several studies indicating that obesity is a significant problem within the pediatric population. According to the literature search performed by Baskin and colleagues [18], there are few published studies of interventions designed to prevent or treat obesity among African American children and adolescents. Although studies have been conducted to evaluate the effectiveness of treatment programs, few were found to be successful. Even fewer studies were found on school-based approaches, and the emphasis in most of these studies was prevention rather than the actual treatment of obesity. School-based programs designed to reduce obesity have been more difficult to implement and thus less frequently undertaken [19].

Programs such as "Gimme 5," "Planet Earth," and "Catch" have all focused on prevention of obesity. The emphasis in these programs was to improve nutrition and fitness. These programs were designed to use disciplines within the school, and encouraged parental involvement. They did not address the treatment of those who were already overweight or obese [20].

SUCCESSFUL SCHOOL-BASED PROGRAMS

A study using a school-based approach to the treatment of obesity was conducted in 1984 and was based on the "Know Your Body" health education program. Postintervention measurements indicated that 51% of the experimental group students lost weight compared with 16% of the students in the control group [19]. Another school-based program entitled "Planet Health" was tested in ten public schools in Massachusetts. The researchers found that the prevalence of obesity among girls in the intervention schools was reduced compared with obesity among girls in the control schools. No difference was found among the boys in the experimental and control groups [21]. A final study, "Dance for Health," was designed for low-income African American and Hispanic students. The program consisted of dance-oriented physical activity and health education. Girls receiving the intervention had a significantly greater change in body mass index (BMI) than did girls in the control group. Findings for the boys were not statistically significant [22].

EXAMPLE OF A MODEL PROGRAM TO TREAT OVERWEIGHT ADOLESCENTS

Obesity rates in the state of Louisiana have risen to epidemic proportions. The Behavioral Risk Factor Surveillance System ranked Louisiana as the state with the fourth highest prevalence of obesity in the United States, at 25.5% [23]. African Americans living in Louisiana had the highest prevalence of obesity, at 35.1% [23]. In response to the rising obesity rates, the Louisiana Legislature created the Louisiana Council on Obesity Prevention and Management. The council includes professionals in the fields of health and education, all dedicated to addressing the worsening problems of obesity in the state [24]. Among other recommendations, the Council has recommended programs targeted at youth.

Weight loss programs through local organizations and community groups do exist in certain areas of the state. However, many young people are unable to attend these programs for various reasons, including cost, transportation difficulties, and lack of parental involvement. It was felt that a school-based program in the form of an alternative physical education class, offered free of charge, would make weight management accessible to more at-risk students. Needs assessments to determine accessibility and acceptability of the program included informal discussions with students who stated that they would be interested in a school-based program.

It was decided that the weight management program would be piloted at a school that housed a school-based health center (SBHC). Health Care Centers in Schools operates eight school-based health centers in Baton Rouge. Four of the health centers are located in area high schools, three are situated in middle schools, and one is in an elementary school setting. All sites employ a full-time social worker and clinic coordinator. Each high school is staffed with a full-time nurse practitioner. The remainder of the sites are each staffed with a full-time registered nurse and part-time nurse practitioner and physician. The centers offer preventive and acute care services to their respective student populations.

Observations by SBHC personnel at one of the middle schools, enrolling sixth to eighth grade students, suggested that there were many overweight students. The BMI, a measure of weight relative to height, was calculated on 279 students enrolled in the health center. For ease of calculation, the CDC's Web-based BMI calculator (www.cdc.gov) was used. Once the BMI was calculated, it was then plotted on a BMI growth chart for children. These growth charts represent the normal ranges for age and height and are also available for download from the CDC site. The CDC guidelines for children aged 6 to 19 years were followed so that a BMI that fell in the 85th to 94th percentile indicated a child "at risk for overweight." *Overweight* or *obesity* was defined as at or above the sex- and age-specific 95th percentile of BMI based on CDC Growth Charts [18]. Some researchers use the term "childhood obesity," whereas others feel the term may be too stigmatizing when describing children.

Within the group of 279 children, 25% were found to be at or above the 95th percentile and considered overweight or obese. Thirteen percent had BMIs that put them in the category of being "at risk for becoming overweight." It was decided that given the number of overweight adolescents, this school would serve as the intervention site. The racial mix at this site was 99% African American and 1% non-Hispanic White. Another school similar in numbers, racial ethnicity, and obesity rates was chosen for the control site.

Once the need for the intervention was established, the next step was to solicit the support of various people and organizations. The support of the SBHC staff and administration, physical education teachers, principal, and parents was essential for the success of the project. A partnership was developed with the Louisiana State University Health Sciences (LSUHSC) Research Program to assist in the research process. A pediatrician, exercise physiologist, and nutritionist, all with experience in the field of obesity management, were asked to serve as consultants for the project. Funding by the Baton Rouge Area Foundation provided the material and equipment needed to operate the intervention for the entire school year.

In the State of Louisiana, physical education classes are mandatory for sixth through eighth grades. Students receive a letter grade for physical education just as they do for academic courses. The research protocol, approved by the Institutional Review Board for the Protection of Human Subjects (IRB) of LSUHSC, stipulated that there could be no grade assigned to the student subjects because participation was voluntary. To forgo the assignment of grades, a waiver was obtained from the Louisiana Board of Elementary and Secondary Education.

Because of scheduling difficulties, the intervention class could only be offered once daily to one grade level of students. To maximize enrollment numbers, the eighth grade was chosen because it had the most children who were overweight. Parents of those children were contacted and given information about the project. They were asked to discuss the project with their child. When both parent and child expressed an interest in the project, an appointment was set up to obtain informed consent from the parent and assent from the child.

The intervention class was called Food & Fitness 101 and met for 1.5 hours every other day for the entire school year. Each class period consisted of a warm-up and stretching period, 25 minutes of aerobic activities, and a cool-down period followed by interactive classroom activities designed to increase nutritional education. In an attempt to further increase activity levels, the participants were given the use of pedometers and earned incentives for "mileage" walked outside of class time. The incentives approved by the IRB included Blue Bayou Water Park passes, zoo passes, skating passes, low-fat smoothie coupons, movie passes, tee shirts, and sweatbands.

The nutritional activities were designed in consultation with the nutrition department of the Louisiana State University Agricultural Center. The classes were taught by Agricultural Center employees and SBHC staff. Emphasis was placed on interactive activities designed to be fun and interesting. For example, students calculated the amount of fat in teaspoons in typical fast food meals. Butter flavored shortening served as fake fat and was used to demonstrate the amount of fat in those meals. In some classes, students actually prepared healthy snacks that they sampled and served to invited guests and parents.

An exercise physiologist and coauthor of *Trim Kids* was consulted regarding safe physical activities for overweight children. She held a training session for health center staff and donated materials in the form of exercise videos and workbooks. The exercise activities of each class period were planned and supervised by SBHC staff.

Ongoing efforts were made to maximize the parental role in the project. Parents were given an open invitation to be present and participate in class. Dietary information was sent home on a regular basis. Parents were also invited to attend special classes in which the students presented materials they had learned in the form of skits and role-playing. The students then prepared healthy snacks and served them to the guests. Parental involvement, unfortunately, was disappointing. Few parents participated in the program despite efforts to engage them.

RESULTS OF THE PROGRAM

There were 33 students invited to participate in the program; 28 students accepted and were enrolled. Through the course of the school year, 15 students withdrew or were withdrawn for various reasons, including expulsion from school, relocation, and class scheduling difficulties. Two students were removed from the class because of repeated behavioral problems.

Ten students logged a total of 220 miles on their pedometers and were rewarded with incentives based on individual miles logged. Several pedometers were lost or damaged early in the program. Every effort was made to replace them as funding became available. Of the 13 students that finished the class, five ended with lower BMIs, for a total weight loss of 33.25 lb (Table 1). There were three students who gained less than 5 lb for the school year. These same students had each gained more than 5 lb the previous school year according to their health center records. Two students gained a significant amount of weight during the course of the program. In reviewing their health center records, it was discovered that they had gained similar amounts of weight for the prior two school years. Among the 14 participants in the control group, three ended with lower BMIs, for a total weight loss of 6.5 lb (Table 1). There were three students who gained less than 5 lb and two students who gained a significant amount of weight during the year.

RECOMMENDATIONS

Despite mixed results, the study demonstrates that it is possible to conduct a weight loss/exercise program in a public school setting of low-income African American children. Lack of randomization, high dropout rates, and small sample size limit generalization. For future replication or validation of this

Table 1
Body mass index and weight change results for intervention and control groups

Subject	Intervention group pre-BMI	Intervention group post-BMI	Intervention group weight change	Control group pre-BMI	Control group post-BMI	Control group weight change
01	30.0	30.8	+4.5 lb			
02	26.9	26.0	−3.0 lb			
03	28.6	29.7	+7.0 lb			
04	23.0	23.5	+0.5 lb			
05	32.5	30.0	−14.5 lb			
07	24.4	24.9	+6.0 lb			
08	26.7	25.7	−2.0 lb			
09	35.3	38.0	+18.5 lb			
11	31.7	32.3	+4.0 lb			
13	44.9	41.6	−13.75 lb			
14	31.8	33.4	+10.0 lb			
15	32.1	35.3	+19.0 lb			
20	28.4	27.6	+0.5 lb			
29				47.4	48.0	+4.0 lb
30				37.2	38.4	+7.0 lb
31				38.5	37.9	−3.5 lb
32				32.0	33.7	+11.0 lb
33				27.2	27.3	+0.75 lb
34				27.6	28.2	+3.0 lb
35				22.8	23.9	+6.0 lb
36				25.8	26.6	+5.0 lb
37				38.6	38.2	−2.0 lb
38				36.7	36.3	+1.0 lb
39				32.3	33.9	+14.0 lb
40				28.1	28.9	+4.5 lb
41				47.4	48.4	+6.0 lb
42				30.2	31.2	+6.0 lb

program, it is recommended that this approach be used at the upper elementary school level because the earlier potentially overweight children are reached, the greater the chance for success.

Instead of using pedometers, which are easily broken or lost, it is advisable to substitute different exercise activities that could be validated by a parent signature. This would encourage more parental involvement and support. Some exercise activities might include playing basketball, walking, swimming, or riding a bicycle. The children could still earn incentives for their exercise activities. A less costly incentive might be colorful beads that could be worn on their shoelaces or in their hair; this would be a desirable incentive for children of this age group. When the student has collected enough beads, they could turn them in for a "free dress day," which would be highly valued by students who must wear uniforms every day, or they could simply continue to collect more beads.

A nutrition education and exercise program could be implemented school-wide for all children regardless of weight. For those elementary schools that do not have regular physical education classes, the components of this program could be integrated into existing classes. For example, nutrition education could be presented in health, science, or reading classes. The reward system using beads or calorie calculations could be a part of math class. Students could calculate their BMI in math or science, providing this was done in a sensitive manner. Key words used in nutrition could be added to the spelling list. Funding for the program might include a schoolwide sale of a recipe book developed by the school featuring healthy recipes submitted by students and their families.

Educators and school administration must make the promotion of healthy lifestyles a priority in their schools to assure that students can learn to their full potential. Students learn better when they are healthy. Children would benefit if schools reduced junk food availability and adopted practices in the school setting that emphasized healthy nutrition and increased activity.

SUMMARY

The national data clearly demonstrates that the incidence of obesity in the adult and pediatric population is on the rise. Overweight children suffer from various health problems and have a significantly higher risk for becoming overweight adults. School-based programs can be effective in helping children lose weight. Although school-based obesity management programs require a great deal of effort and coordination to implement, they provide weight management assistance to children who otherwise may have no access to such programs.

Comprehensive approaches to overweight and obesity among youth need to target individual, family, community, and societal factors that impact on nutrition and exercise. A coordinated federal, state, and local effort that provides needed resources to SBHC can help assure that schools stay in the forefront of obesity prevention and treatment.

Acknowledgments

I want to thank Shannon McNab, MA, and Glenn Jones, PhD, of the LSU Health Sciences Research Program for their encouragement and support. Funding was provided by the Baton Rouge Area Foundation and the Agency for Health Care Research and Quality. The following School-Based Health Center staff contributed in various ways to the project: Marla Breaux, Bambi Pizzolatto, LCSW, Dorothy Pate, RN, Kim Barrow, and Diana Cox. Charman Charles of the LSU Ag Center was instrumental in the coordination and presentation of the nutritional education. Consultants for the project included Melinda Sothern, PhD, Heli Roy, PhD, and Stuart Gordon, MD. Literature search assistance was provided by senior level nursing 484 students from Southeastern Louisiana University under the direction of Cynthia Prestholdt, RN, PhD.

References

[1] Webber LS, Bedimo-Rung AL. The obesity epidemic: incidence and prevalence. J La State Med Soc 2005;156:S3–11.

[2] Healthy People 2010. Leading Health Indicators. Available at: http://healthy people.gov/ Document/html/uih/uih_4.htm. Accessed April 7, 2005.

[3] Brantley PJ, Myers VH, Roy HJ. Environmental and lifestyle influences on obesity. J La State Med Soc 2005;156:S19–25.

[4] West Virginia Bureau of Public Health. Physical activity and health: a report of the Surgeon General: healthy people 2010: physical activity and health objectives. West Virginia Bureau of Public Health; 1996.

[5] Gentile DA, Walsh DA. A normative study of family media habits. J Appl Dev Psychol 2002;23:157–78.

[6] Crespo CJ, Smit E, Troiano RP, et al. Television watching, energy intake, and obesity in US children. Arch Pediatr Adolesc Med 2001;155:360–5.

[7] Bowers DE. Cooking trends echo changing roles of women. Food Rev 2000;23:23–9.

[8] National Restaurant Association. Restaurant Industry Pocket Factbook. Available at: http// www.resturant.org/research/pocket/index.htm. Accessed January 5, 2004.

[9] US Department of Health and Human Services. "The Secretary's Challenge Kick-Off Event" Available at: www.hhs.gov/news/speech/2003/031015.html. Accessed December 19, 2003.

[10] Flegal KM, Carroll MD, Ogden CL, et al. Prevalence and trends in obesity among US adults 1999–2000. JAMA 2002;288:1723–7.

[11] National Center for Health Statistics. Centers for Disease Control and Prevention as of 01/ 14/04. Available at: http://www.cdc.gov/nchs/products/pubs/pubd/hestats/obese/ obse99.htm. Accessed January 14, 2004.

[12] Strauss R, Pollack H. Epidemic increase in childhood overweight, 1986–1998. JAMA 2000;286:2845–8.

[13] Bartlett TB, Lancaster R, New N. Pediatric obesity: use a team approach. The Clinical Advisor 2005;8:22–31.

[14] Strauss RS. Childhood obesity and self-esteem. Available at: http://www.pediatrics.org/ cgi/content/full/105/1/e15. Accessed February 5, 2005.

[15] American Diabetes Association. Type 2 diabetes in children and adolescents. Diabetes Care 2000;23:381–9.

[16] Styne D. Childhood and adolescent obesity. Pediatr Clin North Am 2001;48:823–53.

[17] Brownlee S. Too heavy, too young. Time 2000;159:88–91.

[18] Baskin ML, Ahuwalia HK, Resnicow K. Obesity intervention among African-American children and adolescents. Pediatr Clin North Am 2001;48:1027–39.

[19] Williams C. Prevention and treatment of childhood obesity in a public school setting. Pediatr Ann 1984;13:482–7.

[20] Must A. Morbidity and mortality associated with elevated body weight in children and adolescents. Am J Clin Nutr 1996;63:S445–7.

[21] Gortmaker SL, Peterson K, Wiecha J, et al. Reducing obesity via a school-based interdisciplinary intervention among youth: Planet Health. Arch Pediatr Adolesc Med 1999;153: 409–18.

[22] Flores P. Dance for health: improving fitness in African-American and Hispanic adolescents. Public Health Rep 1995;110:189–93.

[23] Center for Disease Control and Prevention. Behavioral risk factor surveillance system: prevalence data, risk factors and calculated variables 2002. Available at: http:// apps.nccd.cdc.gov/brfss/list.asp?cat=RF&yr=2002&qkey=4409&state=us. 2002. Accessed January 21, 2004.

[24] Udall JN, Moore CV, Norton BA, et al. Special issue: obesity in Louisiana [preface]. J La State Med Soc 2005;156:S3.

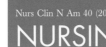

Nurs Clin N Am 40 (2005) 671–679

NURSING CLINICS
OF NORTH AMERICA

The Impact of Violence on Adolescents in Schools: a Case Study on the Role of School-Based Health Centers

Henry J. Perkins, PhD[a],*, Carolyn R. Montford, PsyD[b]

[a]Northwestern University, Counseling and Psychological Services, 633 Emerson, Evanston, IL 60208, USA
[b]Department of Psychiatry, Division of Psychology, Stritch School of Medicine, Loyola University Medical Center, Building 105 Room 1940, 2160 South First Avenue, Maywood, IL 60153, USA

In the aftermath of the tragic school shootings that punctuated the 1990s, national attention focused on the problem of violence among youth. Research efforts were directed at enhancing understanding of the underlying causes of youth violence [1–4] and measuring the effectiveness of various violence prevention programs [5–7]. Other initiatives dealt with the posttraumatic stress that often plagues children who witness or are victims of violence. As reports of violence in schools increased, school districts responded by installing metal detectors, developing zero-tolerance weapons policies, and lobbying for changes in state laws. Other school districts responded to the problem by forging creative partnerships between schools and local government agencies.

School-based health centers (SBHCs) emerged in the late 1960s as a response to concerns about the health care needs of underserved children and adolescents who were often left out of the health care system. Most SBHCs provide an array of primary health care services, such as routine health screenings, immunizations, acute care for common conditions, behavioral risk assessments, and health education on various topics. One of the most important functions of an SBHC is the provision of psychological services for teenagers experiencing depression, adjustment difficulties, substance abuse, and trauma. Data suggest that 25% of visits to a SBHC are for psychological services. SBHCs can also be an important resource for those students affected by violence. Mental health care is an essential service, and preventing and dealing with the aftermath of violence are important components of mental health services.

YOUTH VIOLENCE: AN OVERVIEW OF A NATIONAL PROBLEM
Place of residence, age, race, gender, socioeconomic status, and access to health care play important roles in the ways a person might be impacted by violence.

*Corresponding author. E-mail address: h-perkins@northwestern.edu (H.J. Perkins).

0029-6465/05/$ – see front matter
doi:10.1016/j.cnur.2005.07.004

The burden of violence unfortunately falls on poor and minority children [8]. Although national statistics show that violent crime has declined among adults [9,10], violence among children and adolescents remains a concern. Well over 800,000 young people were reported injured in violent altercations by the end of 2002 [11]. By some estimates, 80% of children and adolescents living in inner-city areas have been exposed to violence, either as witnesses or victims [12]. According to the National Vital Statistics Report 2000, homicide is the second leading cause of death for young people between the ages of 10 and 24 years [13]. The report also noted that for African-Americans between the ages of 15 and 24 years, homicide is the leading cause of death. Homicide is also the second leading cause of death for adolescents and young adults who are Hispanic. In 2000, the homicide rate was 2.5 per 100,000 for white men; 0.9 per 100,000 for white women; 2 per 100,000 for Hispanic women; and 5 per 100,000 for African-American women [13]. Access to firearms has been identified as a major contributing factor to youth homicide. Since 1990, 79% of homicide victims between the ages of 10 and 24 years were killed with firearms [14]. Several national surveys suggest that incidents of violence occur regularly in high schools and that the most common type of violence involves fighting [15]. In 2001, over 2 million students between the ages of 12 and 18 years were victims of nonfatal crimes of violence or theft at school [11]. However, students were safer at schools than they were away from school [11]. In addition, violence victimization rates declined between 1992 and 2001 [16]. A recent Centers for Disease Control and Prevention Youth Risk Behavior Survey found that 9.2% of high school students reported having been injured or threatened with a weapon on school property during the previous year [11].

FACTORS ASSOCIATED WITH YOUTH VIOLENCE

The question of why violence occurs among young people has prompted wide speculation and debate on the possible origins of the problem. Some argue that we live in a violent society and that youth violence is simply a tragic reflection of that fact. Others argue that there has been a decline in those cultural institutions that foster and promote personal qualities such as civility and tolerance. Despite these differing views there does seem to be a consensus that no single explanation, such as violence on television, poverty, or the availability of guns, can adequately account for why young people become violent. One perspective that has stood out for its usefulness in understanding violence, especially lethal violence, is the concept of risk versus protective factors. One of the chief proponents of the idea of considering the balance between risks and resources is James Garbarino, a developmental psychologist who has done extensive research in the area of childhood trauma.

Using an epidemiologic approach, Garbarino [1] examined national crime statistics for 1995 and found that 84% of all United States counties reported no juvenile homicides. Among those counties that reported juvenile homicides for that year, a surprising 25% of juvenile homicides took place in only five cities: Los Angeles, New York, Detroit, Houston, and Chicago. Garbarino observed that factors common to each of these inner-city areas were high rates of unemployment, gang activity, drug dealing, child abuse, racial segregation, and lack of access to health care. Growing up in such "war zone" neighborhoods puts a young person at greater risk [17]. According to Zagar and colleagues [17], an adolescent boy's chances of committing murder were twice as likely if there was a family history of criminal violence and a history of physical abuse, gang membership, and alcohol or other substance abuse.

Research suggests that the odds of a young man killing another person triple if he has a prior arrest record, been diagnosed with a neurologic problem that impairs thinking and feeling, used a weapon, and had difficulties at school [17]. Garbarino asserts that it is the accumulation of multiple risk factors that increases the likelihood of an adolescent being either a victim or a perpetrator of violence. It has been suggested that protective factors, such as a positive home environment, religious involvement, and a positive relationship with school, may lessen the likelihood of at-risk teens committing violent acts [18,19]. These protective factors appear to benefit the individual by aiding problem-solving capabilities, providing mentoring, and supporting prosocial behaviors.

The city of Philadelphia attempted to strengthen bonding with the school as a way of reducing violence among school-aged youth. School officials noted that victims and perpetrators of violent crimes were chronically truant. The school system joined with the juvenile court to identify those individuals who had the worst attendance rates to assist them in getting back in school, thus decreasing their risk of being involved in a violent incident [20].

Although considerable attention has been directed at understanding violence between men, there is evidence indicating that violence between women is also a concern. The Youth Risk Behavior Surveillance survey [11,21] revealed that between 2001 and 2003, the number of adolescent girls who reported having gotten into fights increased for African-American girls and remained essentially the same for Hispanic and European-American girls. The percentages ranged from 29.6% in 2001 to 34% in 2003 for African-Americans girls, and 29.3% in 2001 to 29.5% in 2003 for Hispanic girls. The reported incidence of fighting declined somewhat for European-American girls—from 22.1% in 2001 to 21.7% in 2003. Williams [22] observed that for students of color in particular, underlying causes of fighting are romantic rivalries, flirting, and defending one's honor amidst "he said/she said" rumors.

CASE STUDY—THE ROLE OF A SCHOOL-BASED HEALTH CENTER IN VIOLENCE PREVENTION AND INTERVENTION AT PROTOTYPE HIGH SCHOOL

The following case study is an amalgam of experiences of the authors dealing with violence in a variety of school settings in several states. A case study focusing on a prototype high school can be used to illustrate how SBHC staff, working in collaboration with existing school programs and personnel, can help deal with the effects of violence on schools. The case study high school is located in an older, working class prototype community in a large Northeastern city. The surrounding community had a great deal in common with the "war zone" inner-city areas described by Garbarino. The community was characterized by rising unemployment, crime, gang activity, high rates of substance abuse and HIV/AIDS. Of the 57,000 residents, over 70% were African-American, 10% European-American, and 20% Hispanic. The community had a large percentage of female-headed households and approximately 25% of the population under the age of 14. The community's infant mortality rate (IMR) was twice that of the state average [23]. Excess IMR can be attributable to several factors including poverty, high rates of teen pregnancy, low birth weight, substance abuse and inadequate prenatal care.

.

PROTOTYPE HIGH SCHOOL: THE PERFECT STORM

Prototype High School had an enrollment of just under 2000 students, with 80% of the student body African-American, 12% Hispanic, and the remainder White or Asian. At the time the SBHC opened, lethal violence—most of it gang-related—was a fact of life in the community. Adverse risk factors, such as crime, poverty, poor health care, and the scarcity of strong social institutions in the community, created a veritable "perfect storm" for the occurrence of violence and other social problems. Crime statistics gathered over five years, revealed that 15 adolescents in the community of Suburban High School were murdered. In that same period, 13 young people who had ties to the school were charged with murder or attempted murder.

One of the first challenges the SBHC team confronted was how to become involved in the school's efforts to address violence. The clinical psychologist became the team member to serve as liaison to the school and initiate SBHC violence prevention activities. Initially, it seemed that the SBHC staff was regarded by some teachers and administrators as "outsiders" whose function within the school was uncertain. SBHC staff recognized that establishing a trusting relationship with teachers, parents, and administrators, and clearly defining the SBHC's role was a priority. The psychologist's response was to invite faculty and staff to a series of formal and informal meetings to introduce the types of psychological services that the SBHC could provide. In the course of these meetings the psychologist began to develop a fuller understanding of how the threat of violence impacted students, teachers, parents, school administrators, and the community.

At the conclusion of many formal or informal conversations, one or two teachers approached the psychologist to request a "curbside consultation." Regardless of the reason for the consultation, these encounters invariably turned to a discussion of violence. The teachers shared their individual experiences of violence, feelings of loss, and lack of preparedness to handle such emotionally charged issues. One teacher reported having two students die in violent encounters and felt completely unprepared and overwhelmed by the magnitude of grief she and her students were experiencing. Another teacher reported that while attempting to intervene in a fight between two girls, one of the girls attacked her, and in the ensuing struggle the teacher received several blows to the head. That teacher resigned midyear. A common observation that teachers shared was that students had no place in the school to process their feelings after reports of a violent incident in the community. Teachers reported that anger and overly aggressive behavior were often apparent in the wake of a violent incident and more fighting frequently occurred in the wake of shootings. It was clear that when violence occurred, everyone in the school and the community was affected.

Violence among school-aged youth and young adults is handled in different ways depending on the culture of the school and community, available resources, and the policy preferences of school administrators. Some affluent school districts have well-developed crisis teams with set protocols if a child dies or suffers a serious accident. Other schools do not have well-designed policies and can benefit from the expertise and additional resources of the SBHC team.

When the SBHC opened at Prototype High School, a crisis committee headed by a social worker was in place and included the principal, deans, school nurse, head of security, and teachers. The team relied on a phone tree to alert key school personnel about a violent incident. Unfortunately, notification of an incident seldom moved beyond one or two levels, leaving many people out of the information loop. Prototype High School's policy regarding death notifications called for the principal to announce a student death over the school's public announcement system, and then ask for a minute of prayerful silence. However, in instances where it was perceived that the student who was killed was a member of a gang, no announcement was made for fear of glorifying the death. Following the violent incident, a member of the school's crisis team, usually a social worker, would make an appearance in each of the deceased student's classes. The team member would provide additional information about the student victim. This contact involved little or no processing of student reactions to the death. In cases where the victim or perpetrators were thought to be gang members, fellow students were not excused from class to attend the funeral and no public notification was made in an effort to lessen the impression of a widening gang problem.

Although Prototype High School had no established arrangement for grieving students to process their feelings, teachers and administrators frequently opened their hearts and homes to students who had been touched by violence. On numerous occasions such outpourings of support made a critical difference in assisting students as they coped with a violence-related crisis.

Students of Prototype High School developed their own rituals for coping with the death of their classmates. One of these rituals involved wearing a tee shirt embossed with a picture of the deceased student. Unfortunately, this practice of honoring a dead classmate was used as another way to threaten fellow students with violence by saying, "I'll put your face on a tee shirt." This threat was perhaps the starkest example of the almost commonplace acceptance of violence at the high school in this community.

In neighborhoods where there is frequent exposure to violence, a common set of psychological defense mechanisms may be observed. Some teens react by distancing themselves from any outward display of emotion. This behavior is an attempt to suppress painful feelings associated with loss, and fears regarding their own safety. Coping mechanisms that employ denial and avoidance often make it more difficult for affected individuals to proactively work through their feelings in ways that result in a sense of positive resolution [2].

Among some young people, defense mechanisms such as anger and overly aggressive behaviors are juxtaposed with a sense of fatalism about the inevitability that some people may be killed. This attitude is similar to the concept of learned helplessness popularized by psychologist Martin Seligman [24]. The theory holds that when people are faced with adversity or negative life events they make three types of attributions regarding the cause of the negative event. These attributions reveal an underlying attitude of either pessimism or optimism. A pessimistic attributional style is one in which the individual believes that (1) bad things happen through some fault or characteristic of their own; (2) the cause of a negative event is stable over time or permanent; and (3) the cause affects multiple aspects of their lives. According to the theory of attributional style, individuals who tend to make personal, permanent, and pervasive attributions about the causes of negative life events are more likely to be pessimistic in their outlook on life [24]. This tendency contributes to a sense of being stuck or mired in one's misery. A similar attitude appeared to be prevalent among some individuals at Suburban High School: that violence and loss were inevitable and there was very little that could be done to change that fact.

QUIETING THE STORM THROUGH EFFECTIVE CRISIS INTERVENTION

The SBHC psychologist was invited to join the school's crisis team and immediately became aware of two critical shortcomings: there was no formal written plan in place for responding to off-campus student shootings and there was no established tie with a community crisis team that could provide trained mental health workers to do crisis counseling and referral. The psychologist attempted to bring attention to how the plan could be improved, and volunteered to work on a committee to reformulate the school's crisis plan. The committee consisted of the psychologist and two school social workers. They made the following recommendations:

- Design a crisis intervention plan to include members of the school and community in collaborative partnerships.
- Train staff and faculty to recognize signs of acute stress and depression.
- Provide year-long in-service training on violence and violence prevention.
- Designate a school classroom as a debriefing room where students could meet in small groups with a staff member to process their feelings.
- Use community-based crisis teams.
- Provide life skills training.

The committee's recommendations incorporated features of other intervention and prevention programs with proven success records. These features include involvement of parents, community organizations, and religious institutions; an emphasis on promoting a healthier school climate; instruction on and promotion of conflict resolution skills; and the provision of appropriate mental health services [19,25].

Unfortunately, it wasn't long before the revised crisis plan was put to the test. That test came in the form of a shooting that occurred in the school's parking lot, witnessed by almost a dozen students. A debriefing room had been set aside where small groups of students were able to meet with one of the school's mental health professionals. The goal was to provide triage and risk screening for those students who had been directly exposed to the shooting. Students were screened for acute stress reactions in the form of agitation; anxiety; irritability; feelings of depersonalization or derealization (eg, sense of detachment, out-of-body experience); intense grief reactions; confusion; poor concentration; intrusive thoughts; and physical complaints such as headaches and gastrointestinal upsets.

Students in need of ongoing support were referred to an in-house mental health professional or to local community agencies. The revised plan was useful in that several at-risk students were identified and provided extra support. However, the lack of a sufficient number of trained crisis counselors made it difficult to attend to the needs of all the students. A life skills program was initiated in which the psychologist worked with small groups of six to eight students and focused on topics such as anger management, conflict resolution, communication training, and relationship-building skills. The life skills component was able to reach more students because of the group approach.

Long-term plans for violence prevention and intervention

Another positive outcome of the reorganization of the crises team and SBHC personnel involvement was an increased acknowledgment of the problem of violence coupled with a new sense of hope that things could change. Rather than denying that violence was a problem in the school and community, school administrators embraced it as an important issue. The school's grant-writing team sought and secured a large federal grant to institute a violence prevention program. Community leaders organized a march against violence to demonstrate commitment to change. Church groups, elected officials, and community groups continue to meet to work on solutions. There is renewed interest in community development to attract jobs and businesses. SBHC mental health staff continue to be an integral part of the crises team and are involved in ongoing violence prevention activities.

SUMMARY

The problem of violence among young people is complex and multifaceted, and requires interventions on multiple levels. There is no quick and simple solution. Guns are far too available to young men who in the past may have settled a personal dispute with their fists. Street gangs and the allure of easy drug money offer a perverse sense of family and security to youngsters whose real families struggle against the weight of poverty and unemployment. Violence in the larger society and community spills over into schools and playgrounds. Gun control, combating the drug trade, and addressing the issues of poverty, unemployment, and poor-performing schools are problems that confront our nation as a whole, and as such require a national effort. Concerted national effort is of vital importance if our primary and secondary schools are to remain safe and nurturing environments suitable to prepare our teenagers for the challenges and opportunities that lie beyond their high school years. SBHCs can be an important frontline defense in the provision of crisis intervention services and violence prevention programs. Dealing with violence and its aftermath is hard work for SBHC staff, schools, parents, young people, and the community. However, working collaboratively will help reach the goal of a safe and nurturing school environment that promotes learning.

FURTHER READINGS

UCLA School Mental Health Project. Available at: http://smhp.psych.ucla.edu/.

National Youth Gang Center. Available at: http://www.iir.com/nygc/.

National Institute of Mental Health. Available at: http://www.nimh.nih.gov/.

National Center for Injury Prevention and Control Available at: http://www.cdc.gov/nipc/factsheets/yvfacts.htm.

National School Safety Center. Available at: http://www.nssc1.org/.

National Youth Violence Prevention Research Center. Available at: http://www.safeyouth.org/scripts/index.asp.

Student Pledge Against Gun Violence. Available at: http://www.pledge.org/.

Violence and Injury Control Through Education, Networking and Training on the World Wide Web. Available at: http://www.sph.unc.edu/vincentweb/.

Office of Civil Rights. Available at: http://www.ed.gov/about/offices/list/ocr/index.html.

Division of Adolescent and School Health (DASH). Available at: http://www.cdc.gov/HealthyYouth/index.htm.

References

[1] Garbarino J. Lost boys: why our sons turn violent and how we can save them. New York: Free Press; 1999.

[2] Flaherty L. School violence and the school environment. In: Shafii M, Shafii SL, editors. School violence: assessment, management, prevention. Washington, DC: American Psychiatric Publishing, Inc.; 2001.

[3] Lowry R, Powell KE, Kann L, et al. Weapon-carrying, physical fighting, and fight-related injury among US adolescents. Am J Prev Med 1998;14:122–9.

[4] Winett LB. Constructing violence as a public health problem. Public Health Rep 1998;113: 498–507.

[5] Sheehan K, DiCaru J, LeBailly S, et al. Adapting the gang model: peer mentoring for violence prevention. Pediatrics 1999;104:50–4.

[6] Resnick MA, Bearman PS, Blum RW, et al. Protecting adolescents from harm: findings from the National Longitudinal Study of Adolescent Health. JAMA 1997;278:823–32.

[7] Bender W, McLaughlin P. Violence in the classroom: where we stand. Intervention in School and Clinic 1997;32:196–8.

[8] Rand Corporation. Helping children cope with violence: a school based program that works. Available at: www.rand.org/publications/RB/RB4557-1/-27.2kb. Accessed March 25, 2005.

[9] Mika M. Good news on guns-but not for everyone. JAMA 1998;280:403–4.
[10] National Center for Health Statistics. 1996 Firearm deaths. Hyattsville (MD): National Center for Health Statistics; 1998.
[11] Centers for Disease Control and Prevention. Youth risk behavior surveillance—United States, 2003. Morbidity and Mortality Weekly reports May 21, 2004 Vol . 53, (SS-2). Available at: www.cdc.gov/mmwr/pdf. Accessed March 25, 2005.
[12] Shakoor BH, Chalmers D. Co-victimization of African-American children who witness violence: effects on cognitive, emotional and behavioral development. JAMA 1991;83: 233–8.
[13] Anderson RN, Smith BL. Deaths: leading causes for 2001. Natl Vital Stat Rep 2003;52(9): 1–86.
[14] National Center for Injury Prevention and Control. Youth violence fact sheet. Available at: www.cdc.gov/ncip. Accessed March 25, 2005.
[15] Heaviside S, Rowand C, Williams C, et al. Violence and discipline problems in US public schools: 1996–97 (NCES 98–030). Washington (DC): US Department of Education, National Center for Education Statistics; 1998.
[16] National Center for Educational Statistics. Indicators of School crime and safety, youth violence fact sheet. Available at: www.nces.ed.gov/. Accessed March 25, 2005.
[17] Zagar R, Arbit J, Sylvies R, et al. Homicidal adolescents: a replication. Psychol Rep 1990;67(3):1235–42.
[18] Dryfoos J. Safe passage: making it through adolescence in a risky society. New York: Oxford University Press; 1998.
[19] Johnson DW, Johnson R. Teaching students to be peacemakers. 3rd edition. Edinn (MA): Interaction Book Company; 1995.
[20] Fink PJ. Problems with and solutions for school violence. In: Shafii M, Shafii SL, editors. School violence: assessment, management, prevention. Washington, DC: American Psychiatric Publishing, Inc.; 2001.
[21] Centers for Disease Control and Prevention. Youth risk behavior surveillance—United States, 2001. Morbidity and Mortality Weekly reports 2002; 51(SS-4), 1–64. Available at: www.cdc.gov/mmwr/pdf. Accessed March 25, 2005.
[22] Williams KM. Frontin' it. In: Burstyn JN, Bender G, Casella R, et al, editors. Schooling, violence, and relationships in the 'hood: preventing violence in schools: a challenge to American democracy. Mahwah, NJ: Lawrence Erlbaum Associates, Inc.; 2001.
[23] Illinois Department of Public Health, Illinois Project for Local Assessment of Needs. Available at: http://app.id.idph.state.il.us. Accessed March 25, 2005.
[24] Seligman M. Learned optimism. New York: Pocket Books; 1990.
[25] Jaycox L. Cognitive-behavioral intervention for trauma in schools. Longmont (CO): Sopris West Educational Services; 2003.

ELSEVIER
SAUNDERS

Nurs Clin N Am 40 (2005) 681–688

NURSING CLINICS
OF NORTH AMERICA

STI-HIV Prevention: a Model Program in a School-Based Health Center

Linda Gilliland, PhD, ARNP, CPNP[a],*,
Judith Scully, PhD, RN, CCNS[b]

[a]Total Family Health Care, Clermont, FL, USA
[b]Loyola University Chicago, Niehoff School of Nursing, Chicago, IL, USA

U nhealthy risk-taking behaviors are the primary causes of the morbidity and mortality experienced by adolescents in the United States today. These behaviors include alcohol and drug use; inadequate physical activity; unhealthy dietary behaviors; unintentional injuries and violence; tobacco use; and sexual behaviors that contribute to unintended pregnancy and sexually transmitted diseases, including HIV infection [1]. Many of the unhealthy behaviors that begin in adolescence can lead to continued health problems during the adult years. Sexually transmitted infections (STI) have been called a "hidden epidemic" by the Institute of Medicine and the effects of STI often go unrecognized by the public and health care professionals [2]. Healthy People 2010 outlines goals to reduce the incidence of STI and improve responsible sexual behavior among adolescents [3]. Specifically, Healthy People 2010 targets reducing the proportion of adolescents and young adults with *Chlamydia* infections and increasing the proportion of adolescents in grades 9 to 12 who abstain from sexual intercourse or use condoms if they are currently sexually active [3].

Over 15 million new cases of STI are reported annually in the United States [4]. Almost one fourth of new cases occur in adolescents and the 10 to 19 age group is at the highest risk for acquiring STI [4]. Adolescents and young adults are at higher risk because they are more likely to have more than one sexual partner, engage in unprotected sex, or have sex with partners who have a STI [4].

Prevalence of STI does not parallel self-reports of sexual behaviors or rates of unintended pregnancy. In regard to teenagers and pregnancy, overall in the United States, fewer adolescents are engaging in behaviors that result in pregnancy. Pregnancy and birth rates are declining in the teenage population. In 2001, the percentage of high school students reporting ever having had sexual

*Corresponding author. *E-mail address:* lgillila@bellsouth.net (L. Gilliland).

0029-6465/05/$ – see front matter   © 2005 Elsevier Inc. All rights reserved.
doi:10.1016/j.cnur.2005.07.001   nursing.theclinics.com

intercourse decreased 8.9% from 1999. Similarly, in 2001, the percentage of high school students reporting that they were currently sexually active declined 4.8% in that same period [4]. Rates among boys and girls also differ. Boys are more likely than girls to report having had sexual intercourse. In addition, self-reported sexual intercourse is higher among high school seniors (65%) compared with ninth graders (34%). There also exist major differences in sexual activity among racial and ethnic groups. According to the Centers for Disease Control and Prevention, statistics on adolescents and young adults indicate that non-Hispanic blacks have the highest rates of sexual intercourse (61%), followed by Hispanics (48%) and non-Hispanic whites (43%). Non-Hispanic black youth who are sexually active, however, are the most likely group to use condoms. In addition, since 1993, condom use has increased 13.3% among adolescents who are sexually active [4]. Unfortunately, the use of alcohol and other drugs has increased, which increases the likelihood of adolescents engaging in sexual activity.

There are different prevalence rates for STI among different population subgroups in the United States. Human papilloma virus, trichomoniasis, and *Chlamydia* account for 88% of STI in young people [5], whereas syphilis rates are low in this age group. The infection rates for gonorrhea in all age, racial, and ethnic groups has decreased, but *Chlamydia* is increasing among adolescents and young adults [4]. African Americans have a disproportionately higher incidence rate of *Chlamydia* than other racial and ethnic groups. In 2001, the prevalence of *Chlamydia* infection for non-Hispanic black males in the 15 to 19 age groups was 11 times higher than the rate for non-Hispanic white males. Likewise, the incidence rate for *Chlamydia* for non-Hispanic black females was three times that of Hispanics and seven times that of non-Hispanic whites [4]. *Chlamydia* is more prevalent in females than in males. For example, in one clinic-based study, 30% of female adolescents were diagnosed with *Chlamydia* infections compared with 5% of males. Differences in rates may be caused by differences in the proportion of females who are screened and the fact that females are more likely to have asymptomatic infections. Annual screening and prompt treatment for *Chlamydia* and other STI could help lower these rates among young people in the future.

The higher prevalence of STI among adolescents reflects both risky adolescent sexual behaviors and system barriers to quality STI prevention services in the United States. Adolescents may be more knowledgeable than the general public on some aspects of STI and prevention. However, there are misconceptions and large gaps in knowledge among young people, including those who are sexually active [6]. Even if teenagers may know more than adults do about STI, knowledge levels among both groups is low [6]. Lack of knowledge is only one factor contributing to high STI rates. Adolescents in need of appropriate prevention and reproductive health services often face many barriers. These may include discomfort in discussing reproductive health issues with parents and health care providers, concerns about confidentiality, lack of insurance, lack of transportation, and discomfort with facilities and services not designed for adolescents [7].

SCHOOL-BASED HEALTH CENTERS

School-based health centers (SBHC) were first established in the United States over 25 years ago to improve access to care for low socioeconomic children and ensure that school-aged children receive quality primary health care [8]. SBHC are in a unique position to reduce risky sexual behaviors. Health promotion focusing on reproductive health and STI is an important component of SBHC programs. Unfortunately, public perceptions about SBHC are often at odds with the reality of services provided. For example, when the idea of opening a SBHC is first proposed in a community, some people may equate SBHC services with "passing out condoms" and nothing else. Some community leaders, school administrators, and parents may not be comfortable with the delivery of reproductive health services or the open discussion of sexuality in a school setting. SBHC are usually more comfortable providing in-depth health education or counseling about STI and HIV-AIDS prevention. Depending on state laws, some SBHC prescribe or dispense contraceptives and provide confidential STI treatment services. Other SBHC provide only counseling and education and make referrals to local health departments, hospitals, or community agencies, such as Planned Parenthood. Newly opened SBHC often begin by providing only education and prevention, and some eventually evolve to the provision of contraceptive and reproductive services. The values and preference of the community, school administrators, and parents must always be honored. Currently, about 10% to 18% of visits to SBHC are for reproductive services. The National Assembly for School based Health Care survey of SBHC revealed that 60% provided STI diagnosis and treatment and only about 25% of SBHC dispensed contraception on site [9].

EVALUATION OF SCHOOL-BASED HEALTH CENTER SEXUALLY TRANSMITTED INFECTIONS AND REPRODUCTIVE SERVICES

The literature on the effectiveness of SBHC programs demonstrates that school-based programs have the potential to reduce adolescent risk-taking behavior by delaying initiation of intercourse, reducing the frequency and number of adolescent partners, and increasing the use of condoms or other contraceptives [10,11]. Research has found SBHC deliver significantly more of the recommended preventive health counseling than other sources of care [12]. There is some evidence that SBHC programs that focus on providing family planning services can delay students' initiation of sexual activity [13]. Other studies have explored differences in care provided by a SBHC and a hospital-based pediatric clinic. Data suggest that adolescents with access to SBHC services had significantly more visits for health care maintenance and counseling than adolescents using a pediatric clinic [14]. Adolescents often need to visit a health care provider several times before they feel comfortable in discussing sexual health matters. A standard of care in SBHC is to conduct a behavioral risk assessment on each student and discussion of unhealthy risk behaviors is an integral part of the health center visit. Because of this emphasis on risk reduction and encouraging resilient protective behaviors, students are more likely to discuss their problems and concerns with health care providers at SBHCs.

EXAMPLE OF A PREVENTION AND TREATMENT PROGRAM

Although most SBHC treat STI among their patient population, several have developed specific programs to address prevention of STI and promote reproductive health. One such targeted program was initiated by a Florida SBHC serving a predominantly African American lower socioeconomic neighborhood.

The SBHC was initiated in 1988 with funding from the Robert Wood Johnson Foundation. The SBHC is currently funded by the county hospital through a one half penny sales tax. The staff of the SBHC includes a nurse practitioner, a registered nurse, a licensed social worker, and a receptionist and medical records clerk. A full range of health care services are offered including health promotion, treatment of minor illness and injuries, laboratory services, family planning, STI-HIV testing, and mental health counseling. Every student who visits the SBHC for an acute illness, a physical examination, or mental health services is asked to complete a behavioral risk assessment tool. The American Academy of Pediatrics recommends guidelines for pediatric health care services, and details the content of behavioral risk assessments to obtain appropriate diagnoses and treatment plans [15]. The tool used at the SBHC was modeled on the Guidelines for Adolescent Preventive Services, a tool developed by the American Medical Association [16].

ACTIVITIES TARGETING RISKY SEXUAL BEHAVIORS

Because data revealed that the county is burdened with the highest STI-HIV-AIDS rates in the state [17], the focus is on providing prevention and intervention strategies targeted at reducing STI rates in the high school. Currently, the program uses a two-pronged approach. The first component provides primary health care, which includes identification and treatment of STI and HIV-AIDS and mental health counseling. The second component engages students in prevention programs through the development of a STI and HIV-AIDS website, classroom teaching, an adolescent peer mentoring program, and community involvement.

The SBHC provides a wide variety of STI testing and contraceptive services free to all students enrolled in the health center. Because of the sensitive nature of the services provided, enrollment requires notarized parental consent. The SBHC has a notary on site and parents often come in to sign the consent form. A local social service organization offers confidential HIV testing on site on a regular basis for students enrolled at the SBHC. The nurse practitioner provides other STI testing and reproductive services, including gynecologic examinations. Urine *Chlamydia* testing is available and conducted on all sexually active male and female adolescents. Consistent with national data, the community is experiencing an increased incidence of *Chlamydia* among young persons [17].

The SBHC promotes abstinence first and supports safer sex for adolescents that do not choose abstinence. Various contraceptives are available to adolescents that are sexually active. Free condoms are also available to all enrolled sexually active adolescents. Condom use is also encouraged for those female students choosing hormonal contraceptives. Business cards listing the health center's numbers and other local community agencies are available. The cards provide information on locations for students to receive emergency oral contraception if they have unprotected sex. Emergency oral contraception and counseling are also available to students within 72 hours after unprotected sex for young women enrolled at the SBHC.

Several innovations have been developed to accommodate the large number of students (3000) who could benefit from SBHC services. A unique group physical model was implemented to supplement the regular physical examination performed by primary care providers. On selected days of the school year, group physical examinations are conducted. A system was developed that maximizes the quality and comprehensiveness of the physical examinations and at the same time does not compromise student confidentiality. Health education seminars are conducted in groups, whereas interviews, which include risk assessments, and physical examinations are done individually.

Medical students from the local medical school work with SBHC primary care providers to implement the group physical process. High school students begin the program by attending seminars, which may include topics on diet, exercise, STI, healthy lifestyles, and self-esteem. One station highlights the various programs offered by the SBHC and health education materials are available on health-related topics. Students process through various stations including height and weight, vital signs, vision, blood work, individual physical examinations, and risk assessments. The adolescent risk assessment tool helps determine students' risk status.

Students determined to be at risk for STI-HIV are encouraged to make appointments with the social worker and are invited to attend programs to decrease the likelihood of developing STI-HIV. The social worker provides individual and group counseling and group activity programs and targeted workshops. These include self-esteem workshops to improve students' self-concept. The social worker goes into classrooms on a regular basis to provide education on various topics, such as STI-HIV prevention, self-esteem, stress management, and other mental health subjects. Another program, "Baby Think it Over," is offered annually at the SBHC to adolescent girls determined to be at risk for pregnancy. Participants take home a doll for several weeks and are required to care for the doll as they would an infant. The goal is to point out to students the burdens of child care and discourage students from early pregnancies.

The second prong of the program focuses on prevention and building esteem through developing peer educators and a STI-HIV website. Peer education programs have been shown to be effective in increasing HIV-AIDS awareness and improving condom use [7,18]. Peers are often adolescents' major reference groups and can influence their sexual risk behaviors. Using other adolescents for role modeling and education has been shown to be an effective method to modify adolescent sexual risk behaviors [7,18].

The SBHC staff directs and supervises the peer educators in conjunction with adolescent volunteers. Approximately 50 candidates each year are recruited to be peer educators. They learn about the program by word of mouth, referrals, and classroom presentations and from other peer educators. Students are required to participate in 8 hours of training and testing to prepare them to become peer educators. These trained peer educators lead school activities, which include classroom sessions on STI-HIV, community health resources, communication and negotiation skills to say "no," and safer sex strategies. At these sessions, participants are given a pretest and posttest questionnaire on the subject matter discussed to provide feedback to peer educators on the effectiveness of their teaching. Data from the questionnaires are then used to improve strategies and methods. Peer educators meet regularly to develop new programs and activities, which may include health fairs, speaking at school assemblies, and participating in walk-a-thons in the community. These activities are ways the peer educators get their messages out about abstinence, safer sex, and prevention of STI beyond the classroom setting.

Another way to maximize outreach and reduce risky sexual behaviors is the creation of a STI-HIV website. The goals of the website are to develop adolescent computer skills, provide teenagers with information on STI and HIV, and encourage work skills by giving participating adolescents small stipends. Initial funding for the website was secured from the National Library of Medicine. The peer-mentored website can be accessed at www.makeitrealnow.org.

The website is interactive and student friendly and contains information on the SBHC; basic information on gonorrhea, *Chlamydia*, syphilis, herpes, hepatitis, venereal warts, and HIV-AIDS; statistics on the incidence and prevalence of STI-HIV-AIDS; and links students to different websites to get additional information on STI, safe sex, condom use, and other important health topics. The website also has an HIV-AIDS quiz, with true and false questions, such as "The first system that HIV-AIDS attacks to weaken the body is your nervous system," or "On September 3, 2002, the first cure was found for HIV." Teachers are involved with the website and encourage its use. To encourage widespread use of the website, contests are held throughout the year. Those students who answer the most questions correctly about STI-HIV treatment and prevention receive prizes. Another component of the website is a section on "Ask the Expert," where students are linked to answers to questions on such teenage issues as: What is acne? What causes bad breath? What is ringworm? In 2004, approximately 2000 high school teenagers accessed the website. Each year, new students are enrolled in the program for continual updating and maintenance of the website. This program runs parallel to the peer education program and compliments the program.

SUMMARY

Prevention programs are a valuable component of the comprehensive services offered at SBHCs. Reducing risky adolescent behaviors is an effective way to reduce the morbidity and mortality burden among the school-age population. Health care practitioners providing primary health care for adolescents have the opportunity positively to influence attitudes and behaviors. Programs using peer educators and youth-initiated websites can increase knowledge and self-esteem and help reduce risky sexual behaviors. Over the past 3 years teenage pregnancy rates are down in the community in which the SBHC is located. Rates still are high, however, when compared with other similar communities and the state. New cases and deaths caused by HIV-AIDS were also lowered over the past 3 years, although the number of infections continues to rank third in the nation [16]. Unfortunately, the number of *Chlamydia* infections continues to increase each year [16]. Because many SBHCs provide services beyond traditional primary care, there is great need to support and increase the number of SBHC prevention programs targeted at communities at risk to meet the goals of Healthy People 2010 [3].

References

[1] Department of Health and Human Services. Centers for Disease Control and Prevention. Assessing health risk behaviors among young people: youth risk behavior surveillance system—United States 2003. MMWR 2004;53(SS-2):1–96.

[2] Institute of Medicine. The hidden epidemic. Washington: National Academy Press; 1997.

[3] Department of Health and Human Services, Centers for Disease Control and Prevention. Healthy People 2010: Focus Area 25, STD Progress Review, July 21, 2004. Centers for Disease Control and Prevention (2003) STD Surveillance 2003. Available at: www.cdc.gov/std/stats. Accessed June 5, 2005.

[4] Centers for Disease Control and Prevention, National Center for Chronic Disease Prevention and Health Promotion, Division of Adolescent and School Health, Health Resources and Services Administration, Maternal and Child Health Bureau, Office of Adolescent Health, National Adolescent Health Information Center. Improving the health of adolescents and young adults: a guide for states and communities. Atlanta: American Health Association, N.C. 2004.

[5] Weinstock H, Berman S, Cates W. American Social Health Association/Facts and Answers about STDs: STD statistics; 2004. Available at: www.ashastd.org. Accessed June 5, 2005.

[6] American Social Health Association (ASHA). State of the Nation 2005; challenges facing STD prevention among youth. Research Review & Recommendations. Research Park, NC: ASHA, 2005.

[7] Caron F, Godin G, Otis J, et al. Evaluation of a theoretically based AIDS/STD peer education program on postponing sexual intercourse and on condom use among adolescents attending high school. Health Education Research 2004;19:185–97.

[8] Friedrich MJ. 25 years of school-based health centers. JAMA 1999;28:781–2.

[9] National Assembly for School based Health Care. School based health centers: scope of services 2001–2002. Available at: www.nasbhc.org. Accessed June 5, 2005.

[10] Kirby D, Short L, Collins J, et al. School-based programs to reduce sexual risk behaviors: a review of effectiveness. Public Health Rep 1994;109:339–60.

[11] Kirby D. The impact of schools and school programs upon adolescent sexual behavior. J Sex Res 2002;39:27–33.

[12] Gilliland L. Quality of adolescent preventive health services at school-based health centers compared to usual care. Dissertation: University of Florida, Gainesville, FL. 2005.

[13] Kisker EE, Brown RS. Do school-based health centers improve adolescents access to health care, health status and risk taking behavior? J Adolesc Health 1996;18:335–43.

[14] McHarney-Brown C, Kaufman A. Comparison of adolescent health care provided at a school-based clinic and at a hospital based pediatric clinic. South Med J 1991;84: 1340–2.

[15] Hoekleman RA, Friedman SB, Nelson NM, et al. Primary pediatric care. 2nd edition. Chicago: Mosby Year Book; 1992.

[16] Montalto NJ. Implementing the Guidelines for Adolescent Preventive Services. Am Fam Physician 1998;57:9.

[17] Florida Department of Health. Catch comprehensive assessment for tracking community health for Miami-Dade County, Florida. Tampa, FL: Medegy Healthcare Information Management; 2004.

[18] O'Hara P, Messick BJ, Fichtner RR, et al. A peer-led AIDS prevention program for students in an alternative high school. J Sch Health 1996;66:176–82.

Nurs Clin N Am 40 (2005) 689–697

NURSING CLINICS
OF NORTH AMERICA

ELSEVIER
SAUNDERS

Collaborating with Key School Partners: Triumphs and Challenges

Valerie Webb, MPH[a],*, Brenda Bannor, MEd[b]

[a]Cook County Department of Public Health, 1010 Lake Street, Suite 300, Oak Park, IL 60301, USA
[b]Millennia Consulting, 28 East Jackson, Suite 1700, Chicago, IL 60604, USA

INCREASING NEED FOR COLLABORATION

Problems that affect the health and well-being of communities today are becoming increasingly complex and interrelated, requiring capacities and resources beyond those available through single programs or organizations [1]. This phenomenon is particularly true for the health of our nation's children and youth. Morbidities and mortalities resulting from childhood diseases have been replaced by new health problems based in behavior and lifestyle choices and social determinants such as environmental conditions, housing, and economic status [2]. Poor eating habits, tobacco use, abuse of alcohol and other drugs, physical inactivity, interpersonal violence, unintentional injury, and sexual behaviors that result in disease or pregnancy have been defined as the new social morbidities [3]. These behavioral and health problems, established in childhood or adolescence, generally have their consequences in adulthood, leading to a lifelong struggle with disease risk factors–the main causes of death in America.

In the United States, 54 million young people attend approximately 129,000 schools for about 6 hours of classroom time each day for up to 13 of the most formative years of their lives [4]. Because schools are the only institution that can reach nearly all youth, they can be a pivotal delivery site to address these new social morbidities. Incorporating health into the priorities of a school has the potential to improve the health status of young people and positively impact educational outcomes. The increasing health, social, and economic barriers facing students are inextricably connected to academic performance, often acting as roadblocks to learning. According to *Code Blue: Uniting for Healthier Youth*, a document issued by the American Medical Association and National Association of State Boards of Education, efforts to improve school performance

*Corresponding author. *E-mail address:* vwebb@cookcountygov.com (V. Webb).

0029-6465/05/$ – see front matter
doi:10.1016/j.cnur.2005.07.005

without addressing health are as ill-conceived as focusing on improving health while ignoring education [5].

Schools by themselves do not have the financial or personnel resources to adequately address serious health and social problems [6]. Effectively improving the health and academic performance of students can, however, be accomplished by systematically combining the collective strengths of education, health, and social services. To effectively merge the interests and missions of these systems, professionals from multiple disciplines, such as education, nursing, social work, medicine, public health, and psychology, need to work collaboratively.

SCHOOL-BASED HEALTH CENTERS: MODELS OF COLLABORATION

Over the last 3 decades, school-based health centers (SBHCs) and schools have been working together to address the educational and health needs of our nation's children and youth. SBHCs are located directly in a school or on school property and provide accessible, quality primary health and mental health care and prevention services. SBHCs are typically staffed by an interdisciplinary team of professionals, including, at a minimum, a nurse practitioner, social worker, or psychologist; an office manager; and a medical director who is generally a pediatrician or family practitioner.

SBHC staff routinely interface with professionals from a wide range of disciplines internally as part of the SBHC interdisciplinary team, and externally with school personnel, parents, and community members. The ability to work in a collaborative and coordinated manner is a critical element of each staff member's job. This paradigm is supported by a joint statement issued in 2001 by the National Assembly on School-Based Health Care, the American School Health Association, and the National Association of School Nurses, which states that, "Although multiple health providers in a school setting may have distinctive and complementary functions, funding, and accountability, their objectives are met effectively and efficiently through collaboration" [7].

Successful collaboration can have powerful outcomes. Collaboration involves the exchanging of knowledge, skills, and resources to facilitate the vision and goals that cannot be reached when individual professionals act on their own [1,8]. Collaboration, however, particularly across disciplines and professions, is not an easy task. As Seaburn and colleagues [9] noted, "A culture of collaboration does not just happen. It must be formed and fashioned by many hands." Developing a culture of collaboration between education and health systems is particularly challenging. The diverse and interdisciplinary skills and backgrounds of school and SBHC personnel can bring richness to programming. However, the obligations and priorities of educational institutions and the professional standards and practice expectations of health care can also lead to service overlap and duplication, and misunderstanding between the partners. Other potential challenges to collaboration may include competition for space, supplies, and resources [10].

LESSONS FROM THE FIELD

Interview protocol

This article explores the triumphs and challenges of collaboration between SBHCs and their host schools from the perspective of nurse practitioners. Telephone interviews were conducted with 17 nurse practitioners working in 15 of the 31 SBHCs currently operating in Cook County, Illinois, one of the largest urban areas in the United States. Cook County includes the city of Chicago and 129 suburban municipalities with a population of over 5 million. SBHCs in Cook County predominantly serve low-income students in either poor neighborhoods or communities with large immigrant populations that are new to the United States health care system. Of the 15 SBHCs interviewed, 11 are located in high schools, 3 in elementary schools, and 1 in a middle school. These SBHCs are sponsored by a wide range of organizations, including hospitals, community health centers, universities, social service agencies, and a County Bureau Of Health Services. The length of operation for the 15 SBHCs ranged from 1 to 19 years, with a mean of 8 years. The 17 nurse practitioners identified that they had been in their positions from 3.5 months to 12 years, with a mean of 8 years.

The nurse practitioners were asked a series of questions that surveyed their perceptions of the following: (1) how well their SBHC was integrated into the school environment; (2) their role in the collaboration process; (3) successful strategies that enhanced collaboration with school partners; and (4) obstacles they confronted. The questionnaire design used open-ended questions and Likert scale responses.

Level of integration into the school

Overwhelmingly, respondents felt their SBHCs were well integrated into the school environment. They identified administrators, school nurses, teachers, social workers, building engineers, security personnel, and office staff as the key school players involved with the SBHC. The quality of the relationships with these key players was described by 12 out of 15 (80%) of the nurse practitioners as extremely positive, as illustrated by the following statements:

- "Our principal and assistant principal 'get it' and are huge players and pass this on to the teachers—everything trickles down from them."
- "We depend on our Building Engineers for what we need—garbage collection, clean rooms, installation of bulletin boards and clocks." "I know how well our SBHC is integrated by how clean it is kept!"
- "Our school security personnel come to the health center when we have an emergency. If you build good relationships with them they are on the scene quickly."
- "The office staff let us know the bell schedules and help us with school-related paperwork. They distribute information in teacher's mailboxes and give us access to reports—like attendance."

Collaborative partnerships between the SBHC and the school nurse are critical but have often been characterized as challenging [11]. The relationship between the school nurse and the interviewees in this sample was perceived very positively (nine respondents reported excellent, five very good, and one fair). This positive relationship may have several explanations. As the SBHC movement ages, school nurses are becoming more familiar with this type of health care delivery model and have a clearer understanding of the differentiation between their role and that of the SBHC clinical providers. School nurses may feel more convinced that SBHCs will not supplant school health services but rather supplement them. Also, most of the SBHCs included in the interview cohort are "older centers" (the mean length of operation was 8 years), implying that a tradition of collaboration has been established.

Interviewees were asked to rate how well their SBHCs were achieving the collaborative elements identified in the "Joint Statement on the School Nurse/School-Based Health Center Partnership". These elements include: (1) inclusion of student, family, and school staff; (2) well-defined roles and responsibilities between the school and the SBHC that promote seamless and comprehensive care for students and their families; (3) mutual respect and support for each partner's contribution; (4) cooperative planning and implementation of school health services and programs to promote the health of the student body; (5) joint policies and procedures that ensure the quality and confidentiality of care received by students; (6) information sharing and exchange that protects student privacy and ensures continuity and coordination of care; and (7) a collaborative focus on student academic outcomes [7].

Respondents felt that their SBHCs were doing extremely well in all areas, with the exception of student academic outcomes. Some respondents (2 out of 14) reported that they were successfully contributing to academic outcomes by spending time reviewing report cards with students at SBHC visits and not scheduling health center visits during class time especially on testing days. However, 64% of the interviewees responded that working with the school on improving academic outcomes was difficult because this was not always perceived as the purview of the SBHC. Also, according to one respondent, the complex social and physical problems of students coming to the SBHC often make it difficult to focus on academic concerns. All interviewees did agree that the role of the SBHC relative to academic outcomes was still an "untapped area" that could be enhanced with increased research on the relationship between health and academic performance [12].

Nurse practitioner's role in collaboration

Nurse practitioners were asked to describe the role they played in the collaborative process and their satisfaction with that role. Responses are cross-referenced in Table 1. The role of the nurse practitioner in collaboration varied across sites, ranging from Very Active ("I'm the first line of communication between the school and the SBHC") to Moderately Active ("I would like to expand my role further but time and day-to-day activities don't allow any further involvement") to Not Involved ("I'm the primary care provider for four schools"). The level of involvement depended on various factors: including

Table 1
Relationship between levels of involvement in the collaborative process and satisfaction

Level of involvement in the collaborative process	Satisfied with role	Not satisfied with role
Very active	4	2
Moderately active	5	1
Not involved	1	2

personality or personal preference; availability of administrative and clinical support; and resources. Satisfaction level was not uniformly tied to the level of involvement.

Strategies that advanced collaboration

Interviewees were asked to name one key strategy that was most successful in advancing collaboration between the SBHC and their host school. Several common themes were identified.

Set the stage from the start

Three interviewees mentioned that a planning period was essential to "set the stage for effective collaboration." From their perspectives, it was important that clear structures and policies were established before their SBHC opened because "once we began seeing students, we were too busy to set strategy."

Establish and maintain channels of communication

Most interviewees felt that fostering relationships depended on the attention paid to ongoing communication. Examples of successful strategies included (1) establishing a monthly standing meeting between the SBHC administrator and the assistant principal; (2) having the school designate a project director to work with the SBHC; (3) bringing in experts to meet with the principal and school leadership to discuss health trends; (4) sending out a quarterly newsletter to all school personnel; (5) sitting in the teacher's lounge; and (6) providing a continuous flow of statistics to key players in the school.

Create formal agreements

One nurse practitioner reported that her relationship with the school nurse was strengthened as a result of developing a collaborative agreement that clearly stated their individual roles and responsibilities. Several interviewees felt that at times their host schools have tried to "dump jobs on them that were clearly not appropriate." Other respondents felt that they were able to avoid this "dumping" by having clearly articulated written agreements with the schools, delineating what the health center can and can't do.

Go beyond what is expected

Respondents felt that providing tangible benefits to the school furthered positive collaborative relationships with school personnel. Four interviewees reported that they provided mini-health fairs or appreciation days for teachers.

According to one nurse practitioner, "Providing activities in the SBHC for teachers made them feel at home and see the benefits firsthand. These activities became a doorway to appreciation." Another nurse practitioner felt that becoming a hall monitor enhanced her visibility in the school, leading to improved relationships: "Kids can be unruly and I saw a need for more adult supervision. I asked the principal if it was OK for me to stand in the hallway during passing time. Everyone was very appreciative and seeing the students in another context helped me to get to know them better."

Value the school community

The need to understand and listen to the rhythms of the school community was threaded throughout the interview responses. One interviewee felt it was critical to look at collaboration through the lens of the host school and to "remember that you are an outside agency and the first priority of the school will always be teaching." Several interviewees related strategies that were successful in aligning the SBHC's and the school's mission. "Our principal doesn't let anyone go into the classroom so we developed a lunchroom series of health education activities." Another respondent likened her success in collaborating with the school to being a visitor in someone's house. "I don't go into your house and start touching things without first asking. Before I do anything new in the school, I always make sure I check with the principal or the teachers." Three interviewees felt that hiring staff from within the community promoted collaboration: "Our office manager is a community advocate. She knows so many of the teachers and parents."

Recognize that each school-based health center staff member has a role in collaboration

Interviewees stressed that everyone has a role in the collaboration process. According to one nurse practitioner, "it is important who you hire because each one of your staff makes an impression on the school staff. If one of the staff is mean to a teacher when they ask for a Tylenol it will always be remembered. I still hear stories about how crabby a staff member was—and that was over 12 years ago!"

Barriers to collaboration

Interviewees were asked to identify barriers they have encountered when collaborating with their host schools. Several were generally seen as "bumps in the road" as opposed to "roadblocks."

Individual personalities

Four respondents felt that, even when formal policies and channels of communication are in place, some staff could be territorial and obstructionist. "It is sometimes hard for people to let go of old ideas and to share their turf." When encountering this situation, some SBHC have "waited it out or found other friends." In one case, staff focused their energies on building strong relationships with teachers in a building where there was little support from the principal. Retirement was reported to have healed other difficult relationships.

Staff turnover

Many of the host schools experience high staff turnover among administrators and teachers. According to an analysis of School Board data conducted by *Catalyst* [13], an independent publication that has been covering Chicago school reform since 1989, approximately 30% of teachers new to the Chicago Public Schools—although not necessarily new to teaching—leave within the first 5 years. SBHC policies and procedures have to be explained and sometimes even renegotiated with new staff. Most of the interviewees try to address the issue of teacher turnover through active participation in annual orientation activities.

Lack of resources

SBHCs differ in the amount and type of resources available to them. As a result of increased competition for decreasing public funds, many SBHCs are facing financial challenges, and lack of resources is an ongoing concern. Sponsors asked some centers in this sample to pare back to core medical services, eliminating mental health, health education, and administrative positions [14]. When this curtailing occurs, opportunities to interface with the school may suffer because more responsibility falls on the providers: "I am invited to weekly leadership meetings but can't go because I have no one to cover the SBHC. I am missing an opportunity to remind school staff what we do here and to know what is going on in the school. If we get so busy in the doing we don't get beyond our health center walls. We need to be visible."

Confidentiality

All interviewees stressed that it was critical to establish clear policies and procedures with regard to confidentiality. "This is not an area where we have joint policies—we set the standards." Many respondents reported that setting boundaries in terms of sharing information was not an evolutionary process but rather something clearly defined from the first day they opened. What was evolutionary, however, was the school's ability to fully understand and accept the boundaries. Interviewees recognized that it was necessary to be "firm but respectful." Most interviewees did not see this gradual understanding as a major obstacle and felt that with time and a consistent message, school staff came to respect the SBHC confidentiality policies. In most cases where confidentiality was a major barrier to collaboration, personality was the critical determinant.

The school and the SBHC operate under different regulations relative to confidentiality. The school operates under the Family Educational Rights and Privacy Act, which sets requirements designed to protect the privacy of parents and students. In brief, the law requires a school district to provide a parent access to their child's educational records. SBHCs operate under the Health Insurance Portability and Accountability Act, which sets standards for the protection of client privacy over medical and health information. Schools may feel that they have the right to student medical information, but SBHCs are obligated to respect the confidentiality of clients. These two regulations can result in confusion and misunderstanding if not addressed proactively.

Divergent missions

Sweeping national education reform and increased accountability standards for core academic subjects in today's schools has placed an increasing emphasis on educational outcomes and test scores. Teachers and administrators are, understandably, protective of classroom time and often question the relevance of subject matter or programs that are not considered part of the core curriculum [10]. All SBHCs in the interview cohort have addressed this potential barrier by adjusting their health center access policies to respect the sanctity of instructional time.

SUMMARY

Schools can be a pivotal site for addressing the complex and interrelated health, social, and economic problems affecting our nation's children and youth. These problems require the combined skills and expertise of professionals from multiple disciplines working toward a common goal.

SBHCs are a bridge between education and health, providing site-based primary and preventive health services. An interdisciplinary team often headed by a nurse practitioner routinely interfaces with school personnel. Developing and maintaining strong collaborative relationships is critical to the success of SBHCs.

The lessons learned from 17 nurse practitioners working in SBHCs in Cook County, Illinois, present a body of rich information and experience and can help inform and guide current and future collaborative practices. Collaboration is not an easy task and requires time and nurturing. Sometimes obstacles beyond the nurse practitioner's control, such as difficult personalities and limited resources, make for challenging circumstances. However, as shown by the experiences of the nurse practitioners, effective collaboration is attainable and well worth the effort.

Acknowledgments

The authors wish to thank all the School-Based Health Center nurse practitioners who arranged time in their hectic schedules to be surveyed for this article. Thanks also to Elizabeth Bormann, MPH, and Steven Seweryn, MPH, for their valuable assistance.

References

[1] Lasker RD, Weiss ES. Broadening participation in community problem solving: a multidisciplinary model to support collaborative practice and research. J Urban Health 2003;80: 14–60.
[2] US Department of Health and Human Services. Healthy people 2010. Washington (DC): US Government Printing Office; 2000.
[3] Saunders R, Fee R, Gottlieb NH. Higher education and the health of America's children: collaborating for coordinated school health. Phi Delta Kappan 1999;80:377–82.
[4] Synder T, Hoffman C. Digest of education statistics 2001. National Center for Education Statistics; 2002.
[5] National Commission on the Role of the School and the Community in Improving Adolescent Health. Code blue: uniting for healthier youth; Washington (DC): American Medical Association, National Association of State Boards of Education; 1990.

[6] Wyatt TH, Novak JC. Collaborative partnerships: a critical element in school health programs. Fam Community Health 2000;23:1–11.

[7] American School Health Association, National Assembly on School-Based Health Care, National Association of School Nurses. The role of the school nurse in school-based health centers, position statement. Available at: www.nasn.org: National Association of School Nurses. 2001.

[8] Bronstein LR. A model for interdisciplinary collaboration. Soc Work 2003;48:297–306.

[9] Seaburn DB, Lorenz AD, Gunn WB, et al. Models of collaboration, vol. 1. New York: Basic Books; 1996.

[10] Bannor B. Health integration in community schools. Chicago: Millennia Consulting, LLC; 2003.

[11] Hacker K, Wessel GL. School-based health centers and school nurses: cementing the collaboration. J Sch Health 1998;68:409.

[12] Geierstanger S, Amaral G. School-based health centers and academic performance: what is the intersection? April 2004 Meeting Proceedings. White Paper. Washington, D.C.: National Assembly on School-Based Health Care; 2005.

[13] Catalyst. Voices of Chicago school reform. September 1999: Vol. XI, No.1. Available at: www.catalyst-chicago.org.

[14] Bannor B. School-based health centers in Chicago—current status and challenges for the future. Chicago: Millennia Consulting; 2004.

Nurs Clin N Am 40 (2005) 699–709

NURSING CLINICS
OF NORTH AMERICA

Interdisciplinary Teamwork in a School-Based Health Center

Teresa K. Davis, RNC, APN, MSN, WHNP[a],*,
Carolyn R. Montford, PsyD[b], Carolyn Read, MPH, MSW[a]

[a]Loyola University Chicago, Niehoff School of Nursing, 6525 North Sheridan Road, Chicago, IL 60626, USA
[b]Department of Psychiatry, Division of Psychology, Stritch School of Medicine, Loyola University Medical Center, Building 105 Room 1940, 2160 South First Avenue, Maywood, IL 60153, USA

The goal of school-based health centers (SBHCs) is to provide culturally competent primary, preventive, and mental health care services for students who otherwise may not have access to care. Often, an SBHC is the primary health care provider for students because many adolescents are uninsured or lack access to other health care service providers. At other times, the SBHC works in collaboration with primary care providers and other health professionals to provide health care services for students and their families. Complex health and social problems and changes in professional practice make it impossible to serve clients effectively without collaborating with professionals from other disciplines [1]. One process used in SBHCs to assure that students' needs and concerns are addressed is an interdisciplinary case review (ICR). The ICR is a method of evaluating complex cases with members of the health care team to ensure that the physical and mental health and social needs of students are meeting or exceeding the standard of care.

Bronstein's [1] model of Interdisciplinary Collaboration may be helpful to professionals in understanding the importance of a multidisciplinary approach to complex physical and mental health needs of adolescents. The model identifies interdependence, newly created professional activities, flexibility, collective ownership of goals, and reflection on process as key components of interdisciplinary collaboration. Interdependence refers to the ability of professionals from various disciplines to function independently, facilitated by a clear understanding of roles and respect for another colleague's professional opinions and input. Professionals from various disciplines have unique areas of expertise. However, in an SBHC setting, these individuals often share therapeutic roles because of overlapping responsibilities, limited resources, and preference of adolescents for a particular provider. For example, a student might choose to

*Corresponding author. E-mail address: tkaydavis@msn.com (T.K. Davis).

0029-6465/05/$ – see front matter
doi:10.1016/j.cnur.2005.07.002

talk to a nurse practitioner or a medical assistant rather than to a psychologist or social worker. Similarly, a social worker may be dealing with absenteeism of a diabetic student and will need to refer that student to a nurse practitioner or physician for better management of the condition. To effectively care for students, team members need to focus on the needs of the student and not on the traditional role boundaries of their particular discipline. Interdisciplinary team members must function together in a coordinated manner, communicating and sharing patient care so that the complex comprehensive needs of patients are met [2].

One advantage of teamwork is the collective expertise and knowledge that various disciplines bring to the table. Working together collectively instead of acting independently in the care of students maximizes the expertise of each collaborator [1]. A multidisciplinary approach provides students seeking care at an SBHC with input from professionals who have various areas of expertise. It also helps in making connections to numerous networks and referral sources and facilitates students' goals, which would be difficult to achieve if individual professionals acted on their own. It is important, however, that team members have clear job descriptions and reporting lines. It is also important for team members to discuss how they will interact with one another and what services each member can provide.

Tension, however, is often unavoidable. In the face of disagreement, productive compromise is necessary. People need to be flexible and adaptable as change occurs. "Roles taken should depend not only on a professional's training, but also on the needs of the organization, situation, professional colleagues, client and family" [1].

Collective ownership of goals is another important component of successful collaboration [1,3]. Health professionals who share responsibility for the design, development, and achievement of goals are said to have collective ownership of those goals [1]. The ICR process operates with policies and procedures developed collectively to guide health professionals who are providing care. In addition, SBHC students are empowered and more likely to follow through when they have input into their own plans of care.

Working together to help all students reach optimum health status is an important goal of SBHCs. To increase effectiveness, health professionals must incorporate thoughtful feedback with one another on the successes and failures of the treatment plan. Health professionals can also help students reflect on their own treatment progress, thus teaching them the importance of being involved in their own health care.

TEAM MEMBERS OF A SCHOOL-BASED HEALTH CARE—ROLES AND RESPONSIBILITIES

Each SBHC differs in the number and type of personnel it employs. A center's staff may consist of a nurse practitioner or physician's assistant; physician; registered nurse, dietician; clinical psychologist; social worker; health educator; certified medical assistant; receptionist or office manager; or any combination of personnel depending on the mission of the institution or financial resources. In addition, some SBHCs serve as hands-on clinical training sites for medical, nursing, psychology, and social work students. In these cases, supervising faculty and health science students may also participate in the interdisciplinary review process.

The nurse practitioner is the health care service provider responsible for delivering most of the health care services to students. Most SBHCs employ a nurse practitioner, and some may be staffed by a physician's assistant. Health promotion and disease prevention are valued along with the diagnosis and treatment of acute and chronic conditions. A large component of a nurse practitioner's work is developing a trusting relationship with students so that there is an open sharing about social, emotional, and physical health problems. Risk assessment and reduction are priorities. The nurse practitioner should conduct a comprehensive risk assessment and work with children and adolescents to design a plan of care. Interdisciplinary practice is critical to provide a comprehensive and preventive approach to health care. For example, a nurse practitioner may uncover depression or suicidal thoughts on a risk assessment, requiring a consultation and referral to a clinical psychologist or another provider who has expertise in mental health care. Another student seen by a nurse practitioner may need additional health education, requiring a referral to a health educator or registered nurse. A nurse practitioner also depends heavily on a medical assistant or an office manager to share pertinent information with them from the student's intake process to enhance the delivery of comprehensive care.

In most SBHCs, a collaborating physician provides part-time medical services for students and works closely with a nurse practitioner to determine the appropriate course of treatment for complex medical problems. The physician should be available for consultation during the school day and when the nurse practitioner is on call to provide advice for medical services that are beyond the scope of a nurse practitioner. The physician's role in an SBHC could comprise participating in quality assurance activities that include periodic ICRs, consultations with other providers, and intermittent reviews and updates of protocols. Conducting comprehensive risk assessments during routine physical examinations may be a new skill for some collaborating physicians. Another role for a collaborating physician may be supervising medical students.

If an SBHC has a health educator on staff, the health educator provides health education services for students on an individual basis and in the classroom and leads after-school student groups. Another important aspect of the health educator's role is addressing issues that arise regarding the health of the student body as a whole. Activities may include health education classes, school-wide health fairs, and health forums for parents and school faculty. The health educator is a valuable liaison to teachers and other school staff and can serve on school committees to enhance communication among SBHC staff and school personnel. Health educators may conduct individual risk assessments for the center's patients and work collaboratively with other SBHC personnel. Having a full-time health educator facilitates a true preventive model of health care because the health educator can work outside of the SBHC, in the heart of the school, and in the surrounding community. This arrangement allows the nurse practitioner and other SBHC staff to continue prevention education in a more clinical setting. Although a health educator is considered a strong component of the preventive health care model, the health educator may be perceived more as a luxury than a necessity. Many SBHCs do not have a health educator on staff, in which case the nurse practitioner or other SBHC professionals must assume the outreach role to the school and community.

Many SBHCs employ mental health professionals, including clinical psychologists and social workers, to evaluate students' mental health needs and provide individual, group, family, and crisis counseling. It is estimated that 25% of SBHC visits are for mental health needs [4]. Mental health providers can also provide in-service programs for teachers, parents, and students to foster positive mental health and promote resilience. Programs to reduce violence, promote conflict resolution, and create plans that reduce substance abuse and promote positive self-esteem are all within a clinical psychologist's and social worker's domain. Mental health providers also conduct comprehensive risk assessments and may make referrals to a nurse practitioner or physician for unmet medical needs, or to a health educator for additional health education.

If an SBHC employs a registered nurse, responsibilities may include intakes, triage, medication instruction, health education, and the recording of vital signs and laboratory results. The registered nurse may conduct home visits for children who have complex health problems, and may assist in case management and coordination of referrals and services. The registered nurse may also perform risk assessments and lead health education groups, such as prenatal/childbirth or parenting classes.

The office manager/receptionist, who is often the first team member that a student meets when visiting an SBHC, needs to have a full understanding of SBHC protocols. The office manager/receptionist's duties differ depending on the needs of the SBHC. In some settings, the office manager/receptionist would be responsible for billing, data entry, and general office duties. They could also assist students with enrollment, register them for appointments with appropriate providers, and inform them of the SBHC patient confidentiality policy and the center's services. In other settings, SBHCs employ a certified medical assistant who has a dual role of acting as the office manager and caring for student health needs. The certified medical assistant can perform laboratory tests, in some states can administer immunizations, and may be trained to triage students who present as walk-ins at the SBHC. They could also manage referrals from the school nurse; field questions from parents, school administration, faculty, and the community; inform parents of the center's services; collect parental consent forms; obtain vital signs and height, weight, and body mass index measurements; conduct screening tests for anemia, pregnancy, and sexually transmitted infections (STIs); and alert the appropriate health provider of any pertinent abnormal findings. It is important that this individual be "student friendly" and welcoming so that students do not change their minds about seeking health or mental health care.

INTERDISCIPLINARY CASE REVIEW

ICRs ensure that SBHC students receive all needed services, either at the SBHC or through referrals to outside agencies. ICR also acts as a system to monitor and track high-risk adolescents in an SBHC. The goal of the review is to design a plan of care that assists students in obtaining the highest level of health possible. ICR may include active outreach to students who might otherwise be lost to follow-up. Guidelines for ICR, listed in Box 1, include adhering to the mission and philosophy of the SBHC, operating under the standards of care of each discipline, and establishing policy and procedures for the case review.

Orientation to the interdisciplinary team and a clear understanding of each health professional's role is important to reduce ambiguity and enhance functioning of the health care team. For example, if a nurse practitioner has never worked with a psychologist, the nurse may not understand when to refer a student to a psychologist versus when to refer a student to a social worker or a psychiatrist. To function in a collaborative model of care, it is important to discuss how each team member will interact with one another and what services each will provide. This interaction is particularly necessary during the ICR process, when decisions about coordination of services within the SBHC and school and referrals to outside agencies are made.

The ICR should include all SBHC team members and meet on a regular monthly basis. Students could be referred for an ICR by any member of the

---

Box 1: Interdisciplinary case review process

QA chart audit: see "Medical Chart Audit" form; provider performs general QA chart audit.

Medical issue review: medical provider reviews the chart for medical issues and compliance with standard of care.

Mental health issue review: mental health provider reviews the chart for mental health issues and compliance with standard of care.

Social issue review: medical or mental health provider reviews the chart for social issues and necessary referrals.

Case discussion: interdisciplinary staff discusses the case.

Plan of care: interdisciplinary staff decides the plan of care for the case.

Schedule next case review date or close case.

Case review documentation and follow-up: decide staff who will complete the documentation, send out any reach letters, or complete any referrals.

All routine clinical staff (eg, nurse practitioner, physician, psychologist, medical assistant, health educator, nurse, interns, front office staff) should attend and contribute to the ICR.

health care team when a team member feels a particular case is complex or when a health care team member identifies the need for interdisciplinary input and advice. The plans of care for two to three students could be reviewed monthly. A member of the professional health care staff, usually the nurse practitioner or the clinical psychologist, can coordinate the ICR process. The coordinator could schedule the ICR dates with other members of the SBHC staff and maintain documentation. A reviewer could be assigned to assesses the student's health records and provide a comprehensive history relating to the student, listing any risk reduction interventions that may have been initiated before the ICR meeting. The social, physical health, or mental health problems or concerns recorded in the progress notes can be listed on an ICR form, which may also contain a student's identifying information, diagnosis, and summary of care. The reviewer can verbally present the case to other team members who discuss the case, and can suggest a plan of care, appropriate referrals, and necessary outreach. The student's primary care provider should be designated to discuss the plan of care with the student for feedback and continuity of care. Students' comments need to be communicated to other team members so that adjustments to the plan of care can be made if necessary. The plan of care can then be documented on the ICR with the student's feedback and signed by each team member.

Identifying resiliency factors is also an important component of the ICR process. Members of the team could spend time discussing risk and protective factors that affect the student's progress. Team members should strive to capitalize on protective factors, such as a student's strengths, skills, abilities, and support systems—all of which mitigate risk factors or problems in a student's life.

Each team member plays an important role in the ICR process. Routinely, it is a nurse practitioner who reviews the student's health records, provides the comprehensive history, and initiates risk reduction interventions. The physician provides expert medical review to ensure that the medical management of the patient meets the standard of practice. The health educator provides key information and referral services. The clinical psychologist or social worker could provide mental health expertise and guidance for particular students, act as a referral source for students' other mental health needs, and act as a mental health consultant for SBHC staff.

Other personnel, such as a certified medical assistant, an office manager, or a receptionist can be members of an ICR. Often, the role of ancillary personnel is overlooked in collaborative and interdisciplinary practice. However, participation of team members in the case review and management process can be critical because the medical assistant, office manager, or receptionist may be the provider that a student first encounters at an SBHC. Students will often share personal information with this team member that they do not share with other health providers. According to Papa and colleagues [2], professionals practicing in an interdisciplinary fashion must abandon traditional, hierarchical models in favor of a collaborative model where all team members are viewed as equal and complementary.

CASE STUDY

The ICR team members for this case study consisted of a nurse practitioner, a clinical psychologist, a physician, a health educator, and a medical assistant/office manager. The following case study is a composite of several students' problems/concerns. The names of these students have been changed to protect anonymity.

Identifying information/assessment

Students may enter an SBHC through initial contact with various health care providers. Gloria, aged 16 years, initially made contact with the SBHC's clinical psychologist and presented with symptoms of depression, including insomnia, sad mood, poor concentration, social isolation, fighting, irritability, and multiple diffuse somatic complaints. She stated that she practiced binge–purge behavior, and even more troubling was her endorsement of past suicidal gestures and self-injurious behavior. Her last suicidal gesture occurred when she was 14 years old and involved the ingestion of five to six acetaminophen pills. She related feelings of hopelessness and suicidal ideation, which were occasionally relieved by self-mutilating behavior in the form of cutting.

Gloria viewed herself as fundamentally bad. She felt misunderstood, mistreated, bored, and empty, and struggled with her identity. Gloria experienced her symptoms most acutely when she felt isolated and alone. Lacking adequate social support from friends and family resulted in frantic efforts to avoid being alone. She exhibited a pattern of highly unstable relationships wherein she displayed intense but stormy interpersonal attachments. Gloria showed a tendency toward marked shifts in attitude regarding family, friends, and others, at times expressing great admiration and love (idealization) alternating with intense anger and dislike (devaluation). Thus, Gloria's style of interaction appeared to be that of forming rapid, positive attachments initially, but, in response to ruptures or conflicts, she would switch to the other extreme and angrily accuse the other person of not caring for her at all. She exhibited abandonment fears that seemed to be related to difficulties feeling emotionally connected to important persons during periods of separation. Suicide threats and attempts occurred along with anger at perceived desertion and disappointment.

Social/family history

Gloria lived with her maternal grandmother in a small apartment with multiple extended family members, including six siblings and an uncle. Her biological mother lived nearby. Gloria's family medical history included a mother who had heart disease and a maternal grandmother who had hypertension. Her father lived in another state and his health status was unknown. The Department of Children and Family Services removed Gloria from her family's home because of her mother's drug use and neglect. Gloria reported being sexually abused when she was 9 and 16 years old. Although she reported that she was not currently sexually active, her past sexual history included one partner with whom she used condoms. Gloria had tried tobacco and marijuana and was currently exposed to secondhand smoke at home. She reported that she did not drink alcohol. Gloria received poor to average grades in school and had poor school attendance.

Health history

Gloria reported having had a physical examination on entry into high school, but currently did not have a primary care provider. Her past medical history was negative for any chronic problems, hospitalizations, or surgeries. She reported that she was unsure of the status of her immunizations, including hepatitis B. She took no medications and had no known allergies. Her last dental examination was 1 year prior to her contact with the SBHC and she reported brushing her teeth only in the morning and never flossing. The risk assessment, conducted by the health educator, revealed multiple risk factors, including poor school performance and absenteeism; poor social support and interpersonal relationships; risky sexual behavior; risk for depression and anxiety; history of self-injury and alleged sexual abuse; and family disruption. Nutritionally, she reported regularly skipping breakfast and lunch and eating junk food almost every day, including large amounts of soda. She did not exercise except if she had physical education class at school.

CASE FORMULATION/DIAGNOSIS

Gloria's history and symptoms were consistent with a diagnosis of borderline personality disorder (BPD). The *Diagnostic and Statistical Manual of Mental Disorders, Fourth Edition* does not allow for a formal diagnosis of a personality disorder in individuals younger than 18 years of age, but the diagnosis fit Gloria, who exhibited such features. BPD is characterized by pervasive instability in mood, interpersonal relationships, self-image, and behavior [5]. This instability often disrupts family and work life, long-term planning, and an individual's sense of self-identity. Persons who have BPD suffer from emotional dysregulation and struggle to find effective ways of calming or soothing themselves [6]. There is a high rate of self-injury without suicide intent; however, for severe cases there is a significant rate of suicide attempts and completions [7].

Although no national survey on the prevalence of mental health conditions in adolescence exists, epidemiologic surveys indicate that approximately 20% of adolescents use mental health services. However, it is recognized that there is a large disparity in the adolescent population between those presenting for services and those who are in need of but never identified for treatment.

The statistics on teen depression are sobering. The National Institutes for Mental Health report that one in five children has a mental, behavioral, or emotional problem and that one in ten has a serious emotional problem. In one study of 1710 adolescents, 30% were found to have had at least one current symptom suggestive of a major depression; however, only 2.6% received a diagnosis of depression. Depression, anger management, and poor academic performance are the three top reasons why adolescents seek mental health services [4].

Gloria not only presented with depressive symptoms, she also relieved her hopeless feelings by self-mutilation in the form of cutting. Horrible as it sounds, in the United States today, self-mutilation is a way of coping for many teens. It is estimated that between 1.5% and 2% of adolescents use this type of self-mutilating behavior. Although self-mutilating behavior such as cutting was once found most often in psychiatric populations and associated with significant psychiatric diagnosis, it has become a more common coping mechanism in nonpsychiatric teen populations. It is believed that the increase is related to media exposure on the subject.

Multiple medical issues were also identified for Gloria, including obesity; severe dental caries; decreased hearing and cerumen impaction of the right ear; incomplete hepatitis B vaccination series; and the need for a gynecologic examination to rule out STIs. Gloria's health education needs included comprehensive information on nutrition, physical activity, pregnancy, STI, and HIV/AIDS. Gloria's health problems reflect a disruptive family life, limited positive role models, and a need for closeness and affection from people who care about her.

Course of treatment (plan of care)

Gloria had multiple and complex physical and mental health and educational needs. Through the ICR process, a plan for assisting Gloria with her physical and mental health needs was implemented by members of the health care team. Gloria's case was brought to the ICR seven times during her 18 months as a patient at the SBHC. Typically, a case is reviewed two to four times in 1 year.

It is important to prioritize treatment goals and communicate the plan of care to maintain the course of treatment with other health professionals and various trainees. An important aspect of an SBHC's mission is to empower students such as Gloria to advocate for their own health and mental health needs.

There were several issues that needed to be addressed in Gloria's plan of care. At the ICR meeting it was decided that the clinical psychologist would provide individual psychotherapy focusing on the acquisition of emotional regulation skills in a stable and safe environment. The nurse practitioner would provide medical management for identified medical issues, such as obesity, dental caries, cerumen impaction of the right ear, immunizations, and examinations to rule out STIs. The health educator would address the multiple risk factors that Gloria presented on the initial risk assessment, such as poor nutritional habits; lack of exercise; poor school performance and absenteeism; and poor social support and interpersonal relationships.

Gloria's interaction with the psychologist was one of needing to present her "good self," which is consistent with a borderline personality functioning [6]. This behavior resulted in Gloria's overstating or understating her feelings or needs. To maintain the impression of her "good self," Gloria would often reveal her true feelings in e-mails, written notes, or phone messages, or in discussions with SBHC providers, asking them to share information with the psychologist. On multiple occasions, Gloria left her sessions with the psychologist with the impression that "things were going well," only to send an e-mail or phone message stating she was desperate and thinking of hurting herself. Limit-setting and boundary management became a focal point of therapy. Empathic and caring confrontations were used to assist Gloria in experiencing and tolerating disappointment and frustrations in her interactions with the psychologist and other SBHC staff.

The health care management of Gloria included initiating a weight loss plan with the nurse practitioner and a dietetic intern. Gloria visited the SBHC for over 18 months. In that time, she participated in the health center's healthy cooking class, joined the Walking Club for exercise, and learned about nutrition and how to care for a healthy body. Gloria lost 5 lb while enrolled in the health center's Walking Club. Gloria was referred to the school nurse for a hearing test, which was normal; her ears were checked and the cerumen completely removed by the nurse practitioner; she was referred to and treated by a dentist; and she was given a series of vaccinations, including hepatitis B. Because Gloria had never been tested for STIs and had never had a Papanicolaou test, the nurse practitioner completed a well-woman examination. Gloria's STI/HIV screens and Papanicolaou test were negative. All of Gloria's laboratory results were normal.

The goal was to draw Gloria into a more positive environment and engage her in activities that would help her move toward success. The health educator worked one-on-one with her, helping to educate her on conflict resolution strategies, build positive interpersonal skills, and address issues of nutrition and healthy eating. Gloria's participation in the health center's healthy cooking class fostered positive relationships. At first Gloria participated in the cooking class with a family friend who came in place of her mother. She and her friend worked closely together on cooking projects and shared meals together. This class provided a positive and healthy environment for Gloria to experience. It was a safe place where she could enjoy herself and at the same time work on her relationships with others. Eventually she progressed from being a program participant to being the child care and program assistant. This experience gave her responsibilities for assisting with the set-up and clean-up of the cooking program and wit child care, and helped her develop confidence in herself and recognize that people trusted her and believed in her abilities. Her progress was aided by allowing her to earn respect and prove to herself that she was capable of being a full-fledged team member with health care professionals. The health educator worked closely with Gloria throughout her experience in the cooking program and also referred her to other in-school opportunities that interested her.

Post plan of care/evaluation

The entire team had to be in full agreement as to how to communicate and work with Gloria on a day-to-day basis. Team members set specific and clearly defined rules for Gloria. The psychologist assisted team members so that they were consistent with handling her demands. Gloria exhibited a need to have multiple daily interactions with team members. Therefore, specific guidelines for SBHC use were designed and shared with her to involve her in the decision-making process. It was often necessary for the medical assistant to reiterate and reinforce with Gloria the boundaries set by the SBHC staff. Because she was the first person that Gloria met on entering the SBHC, the medical assistant was critical to enforcing the treatment plan. The entire team also had to be aware of the boundaries to be consistent in their implementation; this is the true essence of interdisciplinary practice and collaboration found in an SBHC.

Gloria visited the SBHC many times over the 18 months to see the nurse practitioner or physician for various acute care and somatic complaints. These visits included back pain, sore throat, rash, chest pain, cold symptoms, and a suspected pregnancy. She was treated symptomatically and no abnormal findings were identified. As is often the case with adolescents, stressors and other emotional issues may present initially in the form of somatic complaints. Therefore, it is important for health providers to "read between the lines" and determine whether the student needs psychological or medical support through team collaboration.

After graduation, Gloria was successfully transferred to an outpatient adolescent clinic where she continues to receive health care and psychotherapy.

SUMMARY

Students who have complex health and mental health issues benefit from various disciplines collaborating with one another through an ICR. The information, perceptions, and knowledge that each team member brings to the ICR process is invaluable. Interdisciplinary teamwork is challenging but necessary in an SBHC where students present complex health care needs. Incorporating a model of care that includes professionals collaborating collectively through a case review process proves successful for most students. Coming together as a team is the first step in developing additional collaborative relationships with families, school personnel, and agencies in the community.

References
[1] Bronstein LR. A model for interdisciplinary collaboration. Soc Work 2003;48(3):1–13.
[2] Papa PA, Rector C, Stone C. Interdisciplinary collaborative training for school-based health professionals. J Sch Health 1998;68(10):412–9.
[3] Mattessich P, Monsey B. Collaboration: what makes it work? 5th edition. St. Paul (MN): Amherst H. Wilder Foundation; 1992.
[4] Illinois Coalition for School Based Health Centers. Mental Health Committee. 2002.
[5] Zanarini MC, Frankenburg FR, DeLuca CJ, et al. The pain of being borderline: dysphoric states specific to borderline personality disorder. Harv Rev Psychiatry 1998;6(4):201–7.
[6] Koerner K, Linehan MM. Research on dialectical behavior therapy for patients with borderline personality disorder. Psychiatr Clin North Am 2000;23(1):151–67.
[7] Soloff PH, Lis JA, Kelly T, et al. Self-mutilation and suicidal behavior in borderline personality disorder. J Personal Disord 1994;8(4):257–67.

Nurs Clin N Am 40 (2005) 711–724

NURSING CLINICS
OF NORTH AMERICA

Evaluation of School-Based Health Center Programs and Services: the Whys and Hows of Demonstrating Program Effectiveness

Diana Hackbarth, RN, PhD, FAAN*, Gail B. Gall, RN, MSN

Loyola University Chicago, Niehoff School Of Nursing, 6526 North Sheridan Road,
Chicago, IL 60626, USA

E valuation and dissemination of the outcomes of school-based health center (SBHC) services is essential for the continual growth and funding of SBHCs in the United States. Since their inception, SBHCs have been practice sites for nurse practitioners and have used interdisciplinary teams to provide care for underserved school-aged children. Early research and evaluation focused on describing the types of services and the quality of care provided. Supporters of SBHCs were anxious to demonstrate that the care provided was "as good as" care delivered in traditional primary care practices. Documentation of program impacts, such as changes in population health indicators or improved academic achievement, has been more elusive. Current evaluation priorities outlined by the National Assembly on School-Based Health Care (NASBHC) include evaluation of mental health services using a new online tool; assessing productivity of SBHC staff; measuring quality; and attempts to link SBHC care with improved academic outcomes. Evaluation priorities of NASBHC can be viewed at www.nasbhc.org.

WHAT IS PROGRAM EVALUATION?

Program evaluation is applied research that asks practical questions and is performed in real-life situations. Evaluators use various quantitative and qualitative methods to gather meaningful data. Choice of methods depend on the evaluation model, the theory base of a particular program, the questions to be answered, and the time, expertise, and resources that can be devoted to evaluation. Rigorous evaluation, using valid methodologies, is needed to monitor quality, provide evidence of program successes, and identify areas for improvement. Evaluation may be conceptualized as a way of making sure that high-quality, evidence-based services are implemented as planned to maximize the

*Corresponding author. *E-mail address*: dhackba@luc.edu (D. Hackbarth).

0029-6465/05/$ – see front matter
doi:10.1016/j.cnur.2005.07.008

potential that program goals and objectives will be met. The ultimate goal of SBHC evaluation is to improve the delivery of services.

WHY EVALUATE SCHOOL-BASED HEALTH CENTER PROGRAMS AND SERVICES?

There are many reasons to evaluate SBHC programs and services. Health care providers and institutions are increasingly required to provide objective data on the effectiveness and efficiency of the services they provide. Collecting information for evaluation is no longer thought of as a burdensome "add on," but rather as an essential component of daily practice. Most SBHCs operate on limited budgets with fewer human and material resources than would be optimal. It makes good sense to identify and use the most effective methods to achieve overall SBHC goals and specific program objectives. Rigorous evaluation followed by modification of program activities based on evaluation feedback is the best way to assure that precious resources are not wasted. In addition, evidence of desired outcomes can be used to advocate for additional resources. Box 1 lists ten reasons to incorporate meaningful, science-based evaluation into all SBHC programs.

Unfortunately, there are also less honorable reasons than those listed in Box 1 that may underpin some evaluations. These reasons could include delaying decisions about faltering programs, providing legitimacy for program decisions that have already been made, or promoting support for a pet program by only evaluating the successful parts and covering up evidence of program failure [1]. A more common human failing is to evaluate a program to meet requirements of sponsors or funders but then do little with the data once they are collected. However, honest evaluation and continual feedback to staff and advisory boards can help SBHCs keep and improve programs that work, discard ineffective ways of doing things, and develop new solutions to new problems.

WHAT RESOURCES ARE THERE TO GUIDE EVALUATION OF SCHOOL-BASED HEALTH CENTER PROGRAMS AND SERVICES?

Requirements for accountability in all aspects of health care have sparked a growing literature on health program evaluation. There are numerous theories, models, and conceptual frameworks that can be used to organize evaluation activities in an SBHC. One of the most widely recognized models is evaluation of structure, process, and outcomes introduced by Avedis Donabedian [2] almost 40 years ago. This model has become a classic. Other models in the health care literature include evaluation of (1) inputs, activities, outputs, and impacts [3]; (2) need, process, outcomes, and efficiency [1]; and (3) equity, effectiveness, and efficiency [4]. Evaluation methods tailored to SBHCs have been compiled in a guidebook [5].

The recent explosion of literature on quality and safety in health care can also be extremely useful for quality improvement and evaluation of outcomes. The Further Readings section lists several popular books that are useful for selecting a model to guide evaluation. Other "how to" resources in the form of

Box 1: Ten reasons to incorporate meaningful science-based evaluation into all SBHC programs

Requirements of federal and state governments, school districts, and grant funders to document that resources were used as intended and specific populations were served

Rules of participation of third-party payers, managed care organizations, Medicaid, and State Child Health Insurance Programs requiring documentation that reimbursable services were provided as specified

Accountability to parents, school boards, SBHC sponsors, and community partners who need assurance that services are being implemented as planned and goals are being met

Demonstration that the SBHC is meeting standards of licensing and accreditation bodies

Monitoring and improvement of the quality of care

Identification of effective programs/interventions that could be enlarged or replicated with other groups, and of activities that are not contributing to program goals that should be modified or discontinued

Provision of timely feedback to staff and program managers so adjustments in programs and daily activities can be made to improve services

Justification for the continued existence of the SBHC and advocacy for more resources at the local, state, and federal level

Provision of data that could be used to seek funding for new programs or initiatives if evaluation identifies gaps in services or groups in the school and community that are not yet being served.

Contribution to the body of nursing and public health research on the effectiveness and efficiency of school-based health care

workbooks, check-off sheets, or step-by-step instructions for evaluation are available free online. For example, the Centers for Disease Control and Prevention (CDC) outlines a process for public health program evaluation and criteria to assure the integrity of evaluation [6,7]. The National United Way promulgates a step-by-step program evaluation template [3]. The W.K. Kellogg Foundation also provides excellent resources that could be used to guide an SBHC evaluation [8,9]. Among the best resources for planning programs and building evaluation methodologies are publications of the NASBHC. NASBHC maintains a Web site (www.nasbhc.org) and list serve that notify members of the latest resources for evidence-based SBHC programs, program design, funding opportunities, and evaluation. The Center for Health and Health Care in Schools (CHHCS), operated by The George Washington University School of Public Health and Health Services, also posts many excellent resources that can be accessed at www.healthinschools.org.

States that use taxpayer dollars to fund SBHCs often maintain Web sites that list required evaluation data that must be collected in order for an SBHC to be funded in their state. Twenty states have Web sites devoted to SBHCs. Some SBHCs that are part of managed care organizations or large hospital systems are required to meet the standards of accreditation of the Joint Commission on the Accreditation of Health Care Organizations or the National Commission on Quality Assurance as primary care sites. Evaluation criteria for ambulatory care/primary care are available on the Web sites of these accrediting organizations (www.jcaho.org and www.ncqa.org). There are numerous professional societies, government agencies, and private organizations that deal with child and adolescent health; mental health; substance abuse; AIDS care; obesity prevention; tobacco use prevention; reproductive health; sexually transmitted infection (STI) prevention and treatment; and other health problems that impact youth. Most of these entities maintain Web sites that post standards of care, the latest evidence-based practice guidelines, and evaluation criteria in their area of interest. The Tobacco Technical Assistance Consortium has one of the best online evaluation templates, called "The Power of Proof: An Evaluation Primer", which can be accessed at www.ttac.org. Although this tutorial is designed to evaluate tobacco control programs, it can easily be adapted to any SBHC prevention or health promotion program. Subscribing to the journals, newsletters, and list serves of these organizations can be extremely helpful when building evaluation strategies into specific SBHC programs.

WHO SHOULD BE ON THE EVALUATION TEAM?

The best evaluations are planned collaboratively at the same time the program is being designed. Collaborative planning can help identify each stakeholder's information needs, delineate resources available for the evaluation, and begin to describe the product to be produced and its intended audiences. The lead evaluator can be the nurse practitioner or any member of the SBHC professional staff versed in program evaluation; an evaluator from a sponsoring or partner organization; or even an outside consultant. SBHC staff, advisory board members, sponsoring agencies/partners, university faculty, funders, parents, and students served by the SBHC can provide valuable input. The evaluation team should be assembled and consulted whenever a new SBHC is planned or new program is contemplated. The evaluation plan should go hand in hand with the program plan. Waiting until after a program is up and running to think about evaluation wastes time and resources. However, it is never too late to evaluate.

DOES THE EVALUATION MODEL MEET STAKEHOLDER NEEDS?

Selection of an evaluation model depends on the needs of stakeholders who will use the evaluation results. SBHC evaluators should select a model that is easy for staff, advisory board members, and funders to understand; helps in organizing the evaluation; and yields the types of data most useful for various stakeholders. For example, federal, state, and school district funders often require very specific evaluation information. These government agencies usually are interested in the qualifications of staff, the physical setup of the SBHC, the demographic description of the population served, the types of service provided, audits of budgets, and documentation that state and federal standards are maintained. In contrast, evaluation data most useful to school administrators might be the number of students served, the number of immunization and school physicals completed, and whether or not the SBHC helped reduce absentee rates. These evaluation data are indicators of the resources and structure of the SBHC, processes of care, and short-term outcomes. These data can be most readily obtained by the use of a well-designed management information system (MIS) that yields quarterly and annual reports on SBHC activities.

Managers and staff often have different needs for evaluation data. Clinicians want to know if they are doing a good job, how they can improve quality, and what can be done to facilitate better workflow. Monitoring the implementation of evidence-based practice guidelines, benchmarking, and continual quality improvement methodologies can often answer the evaluation questions most important to professional staff. Private foundations that fund demonstration projects targeted at risk behaviors are often interested in the documentation of program impacts and the cost per level of outcomes achieved. This type of evaluation requires a more complex evaluation strategy. Expert consultation or the assistance of university faculty and graduate students who have evaluation research expertise would be essential.

EVALUATION OF NEED—IS THERE A NEED FOR SCHOOL-BASED HEALTH CENTER PROGRAMS AND SERVICES?

The model of evaluation of need, process, outcomes, and efficiency [1] is one of the easiest to apply to SBHC programs and services. The model emphasizes the importance of needs assessment before planning or implementing any human service program. Evaluation of need asks the question "what services are needed in this school age population?" Or, given the need for these services, "how can the services be designed to be culturally appropriate and effective for the persons we wish to serve?" A well-conducted needs assessment is often required by potential funders as part of the grant submission process.

Use of various techniques to get the necessary needs assessment data is recommended [1]. A needs assessment should start with the gathering of information on the demographic and socioeconomic characteristics of the community, and risk factors and health status indices of the target population. These data may be available from existing sources. For example, census data on communities, health statistics complied by local or state health departments, and reports generated by the school district on characteristics or needs of the school-aged population are publicly available data. Some schools regularly participate in the Youth Risk Behavior Surveillance System [10]. These aggregate data on self-reported risk behaviors are available by state and city. Some states publish a "school report card" that includes individual school data on academic achievement, the percent of students who have English as a second language, and the number of students who qualify for the Federal School lunch program—an indicator of low income.

Sometimes it is necessary to do an anonymous survey in a target school when no other data are available on health status, risk behaviors, access to primary care services, or the prevalence of chronic illnesses such as asthma or diabetes. Surveys may be conducted with parents, teachers, and school staff or with the students who will be served, with permission of school authorities and following school policies. Respondents can also be asked what they believe are the greatest health care needs and what types of service they would find acceptable. Community preference and norms on sensitive issues, such as reproductive health and the dispensing of birth control in the school, may also need to be included in the needs assessment.

The second logical step in evaluating need is a resource inventory to assess which programs and services are already in place in the school and community. This process will help identify any gaps in services that could be filled by the SBHC. These data may be available from community Web sites, community resource guides, or publications of local health care providers. However, the presence of hospitals, health maintenance organizations, primary care providers, dentists, or mental health services in a community is not an indication of accessibility or use by the target population.

Key informants, who have the knowledge and ability to report on school and community needs, can provide valuable input. They could include health care providers in the community; business and community leaders; clergy; parents and teachers in the PTA; the school nurse; school administrators; and service providers such as social workers, police, and operators of youth programs. Interviews can be conducted in person, by telephone, or by a mailed survey. Key informants, especially those of the same ethnic/cultural group as the target population, can often provide unique insights into the needs and wants of a particular group.

Other needs assessment methodologies include small group meetings or focus groups. In a focus group, six to ten similar people are brought together for about an hour to talk about their perception of needs and the types of services that they think would be most helpful for the school population. Focus groups should be homogenous so all participants feel comfortable and free to express their opinion. One focus group could be conducted with parents, a separate focus group with high school students, and a third with faculty and administrators from the target school.

Use of various methods, including input from many stakeholders, is the best way to get an accurate picture of the need for a program or service. The target population may want or need a different type of service than originally envisioned, which is important to know before planning begins. An added advantage of a comprehensive needs assessment is that data obtained can be used as a baseline for later comparisons. In addition, many of the same data gathering techniques are appropriate to use in obtaining information for program evaluation once the program is up and running.

DESIGNING SCHOOL-BASED HEALTH CENTER PROGRAMS AND SERVICES—WHAT'S THE PLAN?

Once the needs assessment is completed, SBHC programs can be planned to meet identified needs and achieve specific outcomes. A program plan starts with the overall goals, lists specific objectives, and then delineates the resources and activities needed to achieve each objective. Short- and long-term outcomes, estimates of costs, and required resources must be specified. Mechanisms for evaluation should be incorporated into the program plan. Sometimes it is helpful to diagram the proposed program in a flow chart to visually outline program flow. The program could be depicted in terms of resources needed to support the program, processes that will occur during program delivery, and expected outcomes. The W.K. Kellogg Foundation uses the term "logic model" to describe a visual way to conceptualize the underlying relationships between program resources or inputs, program activities, outputs, outcomes (specific changes), and impacts (long-term changes) [9]. The idea is to create a picture of how the program should work. The term *logic model* may also be used to describe a diagram that depicts links between the underlying theory base of a program and program components or activities [11] . The more clearly the relationship between goals, objectives, program activities, and desired outcomes are articulated in the program design, the easier it is to evaluate the program. Programs with fuzzy goals, diffuse activities, and global outcome statements may not be evaluable.

To be effective, SBHC programs should be based on theories or models that can explain or predict the relationship between particular interventions and observed outcomes. The theory base or model that guides programs should be clearly articulated in the mission statement of the SBHC or spelled out in the design of particular interventions. For example, some school of nursing–sponsored SBHCs may base care delivery on a wellness model or holistic nursing theory. Other SBHCs affiliated with a hospital or academic health center may deliver primary care using a medical or clinical model. SBHCs sponsored by health departments may design interventions based on disease prevention/health promotion models such as the Health Belief Model [12,13], the Health Promotion Model [14], or any one of several new and emerging theories of health behavior change [15,16]. Mental health programs could have a theory base grounded in psychiatry, psychology, family therapy, or a community mental health framework. Unfortunately, some SBHCs have not articulated the theory base for interventions nor have they diagramed programs using a flow chart or logic model. Lack of clarity makes evaluation more difficult.

DESIGNING EVALUATIONS TO MATCH THE PROGRAM—HOW SHOULD WE DO THIS?

The evaluation design should be compatible with the theory base, activities, and desired outcomes of the program. For example, a mental health program based on a psychiatric model might be judged based on the number of students who have a particular diagnosis who received psychotherapy and medications that reduced dysphoric symptoms during a particular timeframe. In contrast, a SBHC mental health program guided by a community mental health/prevention model might be evaluated based on how many adolescents in the school were reached by a peer violence prevention program and how many potentially violent situations were successfully peer-mediated. Similarly, if a tobacco cessation program uses the Transtheortical Model of Health Behavior Change, which posits five stages of change for health behaviors, the evaluation would need to assess how many participants moved to a stage closer to quitting and how many attempted and actually quit [17,18]. Collecting the necessary data for evaluation can be most readily accomplished by including mechanisms for evaluation into the overall SBHC operational plan and incorporating evaluation into each specific program.

HOW CAN WE ASSURE THE INTEGRITY OF THE EVALUATION?

It is imperative that evaluations of SBHC programs are performed properly. The American Evaluation Association [19] and the CDC have promulgated guidelines to help assure that program evaluations are conducted in an ethical manner and yield information that is useful for program improvement. CDC guidelines list four criteria or standards for evaluation [6,7]:

Utility: will the evaluation produce information that is useful?
Feasibility: is it likely that the evaluation can be performed as planned?
Propriety: can the evaluation be performed according to all legal and ethical standards of program evaluation?
Accuracy: will the evaluation provide valid and reliable data?

EVALUATION OF PROCESS/IMPLEMENTATION—ARE WE DOING WHAT WE SHOULD BE DOING?

Evaluation of process asks the question, "to what extent has the program been implemented as planned?" Evaluation of process documents if the desired resources are in place, monitors daily implementation, and provides feedback to program planners and staff so corrections can be made. For example, what percent of students in the school is enrolled in the SBHC? Are qualified staff in place, trained, and delivering services? Are policies and procedures that meet standards of care in place? Is the advisory board functional? Is the referral system working so that appointments with outside providers are kept? Are staff actually following procedures? How long is the waiting time during peak usage hours? How much staff time is wasted when students don't show up for scheduled appointments? What does the quality improvement protocol indicate about services? Another important process question is who exactly is using the SBHC services and are they the designated target population? For example, students who have English as a second language may not be using SBHC services because there are no providers who speak their language. Sometimes certain groups of parents may not fill out the paperwork to enroll their children despite their lack of health insurance or access to primary care. The question of who is being served is the "equity question" [4].

Sources of data to answer process/implementation questions include monthly and quarterly reports from the SBHC MIS; program records; chart audits; quality assurance reports; feedback from staff; minutes of team meetings; feedback from parents, teachers, and administrators; analysis of anonymous satisfaction surveys completed by SBHC users; surveys of community partners; and focused assessments of characteristics of students who are enrolled compared with the school population that is not enrolled. Some indicators, such as the number of SBHC visits per month, could be considered as either a process indicator of program use or as short-term outcome, depending on the model of evaluation used. The ultimate goal of evaluating process is to compare the program plan with what is actually occurring to see if the plan is being followed and progress is being made toward achievement of objectives.

EVALUATION OF OUTCOMES—DID THE PROGRAM ACHIEVE OBJECTIVES?

Evaluation of outcomes asks the questions, "how do the outcomes we are achieving compare with our predetermined goals and objectives and the standards of our accrediting bodies?" and "how did our program impact the target population?" A difficult question to answer is how much confidence there is in attributing the impacts observed to the SBHC program; this is an issue of internal validity. Did the intervention actually cause the outcome? Another type of outcome question deals with external validity—can the results of the SBHC program evaluation be generalized to other similar groups? Desirable SBHC outcomes that can be measured include changes in morbidity rates in the target population enrolled in SBHC; overall increases in school attendance; decreases in absences among those who have chronic illness; changes in use rates for preventable conditions, such as visits to the emergency department among children who have asthma; changes in costs or resource use; and documented changes in risk behaviors, such as decreases in smoking or increases in seatbelt or helmet use. Global goals such as "good health," "risks avoided," or "better school achievement" are extremely difficult to assess and attribute to a particular SBHC program.

It is often helpful to identify indicators of short-term, intermediate, and long-term outcomes of SBHC programs. These constructs are sometimes also referred to as proximal and distal outcomes or impacts. Unfortunately, there is not always agreement on what constitutes a short-term or intermediate outcome and what may be considered a long-term or distal outcome of a particular program. For example, changes in health knowledge, attitudes, resistance skills, or performance in role-playing situations could be considered proximal or short-term outcomes of an intervention designed to prevent risky sexual behaviors. Self-reported behavior change, such as condom use, could be an intermediate outcome. Other indicators, such as reductions in STI disease rates or teen pregnancy rates, would be considered distal outcomes or program impacts.

Scientifically valid evaluation studies of SBHC programs have appeared in peer-reviewed journals and are summarized periodically by The Center for Health and Health Care in Schools at www.healthinschools.org [20]. However, establishing causal links between SBHC programs and distal outcomes, such as increases in school achievement, remain problematic [21]. In the earlier example describing a health promotion program designed to reduce risky sexual behaviors, it would be difficult to link a particular prevention intervention to specific behavior changes that then lead to enhanced health status in the population. STI and pregnancy rates among adolescents are decreasing nationally for various reasons that may or may not be related to any one intervention [22].

Unintended outcomes should also be monitored. For example, having an open door policy in a mental health program may be a positive approach but could result in a small cohort of young people who visit the SBHC almost daily and use an inordinate amount of services. Drug and alcohol prevention programs delivered to elementary school populations may be appropriate for some more mature students but have the unintended side effect of introducing less mature students to a world they may have not yet considered.

EVALUATION OF EFFICIENCY—WHAT DID IT COST?

Evaluation of efficiency answers questions related to the effective use of resources and the costs of programs. Types of questions that can be answered include: have funds been spent for the intended purposes? Does the SBHC program achieve various outcomes at a reasonable cost per outcome? Does the SBHC program achieve the same or better levels of success as other programs costing the same or less? And finally, is it possible to assign a dollar value to the intended and unintended outcomes of the program? That is, what are the costs verses the benefits of the SBHC program?

Efficiency questions can be addressed by careful cost accounting that assigns costs to the appropriate program component. For example, how many hours does the health educator spend preparing and delivering group health promotion intervention to encourage elementary school children to wash their hands before meals? How many students were reached by these interventions and, of those, how many could perform a return demonstration of proper hand washing methods? How many actually changed their behaviors when observed before lunch? Similarly, how much does it cost the SBHC to perform each sports physical when staff time in scheduling, getting consent forms signed, rescheduling missed appointments, and filing paperwork for reimbursement is calculated? It is also possible to calculate the cost of screening programs based on the actual number of new cases identified in the population. The US Preventive Task Force publishes recommendations and evaluates the efficacy of various screening and prevention interventions [23]. This information can be helpful when considering the efficiency of screening programs likely to be offered in schools.

HOW CAN WE ASSURE EVALUATION INFORMATION IS USED TO IMPROVE PROGRAMS?

Once the evaluation is complete, results can be shared with stakeholders in various formats designed to meet each stakeholder's information needs. The goal is to increase the chances that evaluation data will be used for program improvement. All persons who contributed to the evaluation should be included in the reporting process. People want to know their voice was heard and what they said will make a difference. Nurse practitioners and clinical staff may prefer a report at their monthly meeting so they can discuss findings and begin to plan what changes need to be made. Managers often also want to meet separately to think through possible courses of action. Advisory board members, community partners, and school administrators might prefer a formal written document and a PowerPoint presentation and then additional meetings to discuss recommendations. Parents and teachers would likely want to hear an annual report at a PTA meeting. Students involved in the evaluation would appreciate a pizza party and discussion of how their suggestions have been incorporated. Sponsors and funders usually expect to see evaluation results documented in written reports that also contain specific plans to improve, modify, or discontinue programs based on evaluation findings.

WHAT LAWS GOVERN ACCESS TO EDUCATION AND HEALTH INFORMATION?

There are several federal and various state laws that must be considered when accessing education or health records in schools. The Family Educational Rights and Privacy Act (FERPA) protects the privacy of student education records. Schools must obtain written permission from parents, or students if they are 18 or older, to release information from a student's educational records. US Department of Education rules allow exceptions for organizations conducting studies on behalf of the school [24]. SBHC evaluators should be familiar with FERPA regulations and work closely with the school's designated FERPA compliance manager. Aggregate data displaying the school's test scores or other indicators of achievement are public information and may be used for evaluation.

The federal Health Insurance Portability and Accountability Act of 1996 (HIPPA) regulates the privacy of protected health information [25]. Individually identifiable health information is protected, but deidentified health information is not. For example, a chart audit by SBHC clinical staff as part of quality improvement activities/program evaluation would not violate HIPPA rules as long as data recorded did not identify individuals. However, evaluators or researchers from outside the SBHC would not be allowed to access health records with names attached. Rules for researchers dealing with private health information can be accessed on the Department of Health and Human Services Web site (www.hhs.gov/ocr/privacy). SBHC personnel should be familiar with HIPPA regulations and follow all rules on protecting privacy.

IS IT INTERNAL EVALUATION OR RESEARCH WITH HUMAN SUBJECTS?

The Office of Human Subjects Research at the Department of Health and Human Services (DHHS) publishes rules that govern research and outline protections for human subjects under the "Common Rule". *Research* is defined as a systematic investigation designed to contribute to generalizable knowledge. *Human subjects* are living individuals with whom the researcher interacts or obtains identifiable private information. Six categories of research are exempt from federal regulatory requirements [26]. Sources of data and procedures used for many program evaluations often fit into one of these six categories. Evaluations should never violate human rights outlined in DHHS rules. If the evaluation team thinks that a proposed evaluation protocol may meet the criteria for research on human subjects, or results of the evaluation may generate new scientific knowledge that is generalizable and could be presented at scholarly meetings or published, then all appropriate procedures for research on human subjects should be followed. These procedures include submitting the research/evaluation protocol to an Institutional Review Board (IRB) for the Protection of Human Subjects before any data is collected. Special rules are in place for research involving minors. Parental consent and minors' assent are required for minors to participate or when any identifiable health information about a child is gathered [26]. Consultation with school administrators is also important when conducting research and evaluation in schools. Some larger school districts may have a mechanism for reviewing research on human subjects. If they do not, SBHC evaluators should contact a community partner, such as a hospital, university, or academic health center and consult with the research compliance officer for IRB procedures. It is important to understand that it is not the evaluation team that decides the level of risk of a particular research project; that is the role of the IRB.

SUMMARY

Evaluation is expected by funders, community partners, school administrators, advisory boards, and consumers. Evaluation should be considered an integral part of all SBHC programs and services. There are numerous models and theories to guide evaluation. The type of evaluation depends on the information needs of all stakeholders and the time, expertise, and resources available for evaluation. Collaboration will be more likely to yield useful evaluation results. There are many texts and online resources that can inform SBHC program evaluation activities. One useful evaluation model outlines the questions that can be answered by evaluation of need, process, outcome, and efficiency. Evaluators should also pay attention to evaluation of equity to be sure that those who truly need to program are being served. Evaluations should be performed in an ethical manner. All regulations involving research on human subjects and access to health and educational records must be scrupulously followed. Results of evaluations should be shared with all stakeholders to maximize the chances that feedback will be used for program improvement. The ultimate goal of evaluation is to improve SBHC programs and services.

FURTHER READINGS

Aday L, Begley C, Lairson D, et al. Evaluating the medical care health system: effectiveness, efficiency, and equity. Ann Arbor (MI): Health Administration Press; 2004.

Brindis C, Kaplan D, Phipps S. A guidebook for evaluating school-based health centers. Denver (CO): University of Colorado Health Sciences Service Center; 1998.

DiClemente R, Cosby R, Kegler M. Emerging theories of health promotion: practice and research. 1st edition. San Francisco (CA): Josey-Bass; 2002.

Fink A. Evaluation fundamentals: insights into outcomes, effectiveness and quality of health programs. Thousand Oaks (CA): Sage; 2004.

Grembowski D. The practice of health program evaluation. Thousand Oaks (CA): Sage; 2001.

Issel LM. Health program planning and evaluation: a practical, systematic approach for community health. Sudbury (MA): Jones and Bartlett; 2004.

McKenzie J, Neiger B, Smeltzer J. Planning, implementing, and evaluating health promotion programs. 4th edition. San Francisco (CA): Pearson Education Inc.; 2005.

Posavac E, Carey R. Program evaluation: methods and case studies. 6th edition. Upper Saddle River (NJ): Prentice Hall; 2003.

Rossi P, Freeman H, Lipsey M. Evaluation: a systematic approach. 7th edition. Thousand Oaks (CA): Sage; 2004.

Valente T. Evaluating health promotion programs. New York: Oxford University Press; 2002.

References

[1] Posavac E, Carey R. Program evaluation: methods and case studies. 6th edition. Upper Saddle River (NJ): Prentice Hall; 2003.

[2] Donabedian A. An introduction to quality assurance in health care. Oxford (England): Oxford University Press; 2003.

[3] National United Way. Measuring program outcomes: a practical approach. Available at: http://national.unitedway.org/outcomes/resources/mpo/model.cfm. Accessed June 14, 2005.

[4] Aday L, Begley C, Lairson D, et al. Evaluating the Medical care system: effectiveness, efficiency, and equity. Ann Arbor (MI): Health Administration Press; 2004.

[5] Brindis C, Kaplan D, Phipps S. A guidebook for evaluating school-based health centers. Denver (CO): University of Colorado health Sciences Service Center; 1998.

[6] Centers for Disease Control and Prevention. Practical evaluation of public health programs workbook. PHTN Course VC-0017. Available at: www.phppo.cdc.gov/phtn/Pract-Eval/workbook.asp. Accessed May 20, 2005.

[7] Centers for Disease Control and Prevention. Framework for program evaluation in public health. Available at: www.cdc.gov/mmwr/preview/mmwrhtml/rr4811a1.html. Accessed May 20, 2005.

[8] W.K. Kellogg Foundation. Evaluation handbook: philosophy and expectations. Available at: www.wkkf.org/Pubs/tools/evaluation/pub770. Accessed May 21, 2005.

[9] W.K. Kellogg Foundation. Logic model development guide. Available at: www.wkkf.org/Programming/resourceOverview. Accessed 2004.

[10] Youth Risk Behavior Surveillance System–United States 2003 (YRBSS). Available at: www.cdc.gov/yrbss. Accessed June 6, 2005.

[11] Rossi P, Freeman H, Lipsey M. Evaluation: a systematic approach. 7th edition. Thousand Oaks (CA): Sage; 2004.

[12] Eisen M, Zellman G, McAlister A. A health belief model-social learning theory approach to adolescents fertility control: findings from a controlled trial. Health Educ Q 1992;19(2): 249–62.

[13] Becker M. The health belief model and personal health behavior. Health Education Monographs 1974;2(4).

[14] Pender N, Murdaugh C, Parsons MA. Health promotion in nursing practice. 5th edition. Upper Saddle River (NJ): Pearson/Prentice Hall; 2005.

[15] DiClemente R, Cosby R, Kegler M. Emerging theories of health promotion: practice and research. 1st edition. San Francisco (CA): Josey-Bass; 2002.

[16] Glanz K, Rimer B. Theory at a glance: a guide for health promotion practice. Bethesda, MD: National Institutes of Health; 1995. Pub. No. 97-3896.

[17] Prochaska J, Velicer W. The transtheoretical model of health behavior change. Am J Health Promot 1997;12(1):38–48.

[18] Perez C, DiClemente C, Carbonari J. Doing the right thing at the right time? The interaction of stages and processes of change in successful smoking cessation. Health Psychol 1996;15(6):462–8.

[19] The American Evaluation Association. Available at: www.eval.org. Accessed June 10, 2005.

[20] The Center for Health and Health Care in Schools. Available at: www.healthinschools.org. Accessed June 11, 2005.

[21] Gelerstanger SP, Amaral G. School-based health centers and academic performance: what is the intersection? April 2004 Meeting Proceedings. White Paper. Washington, DC: National Assembly on School-Based Health Care; 2005.

[22] Centers for Disease Control and Prevention. Surviellance Summaries May 21, 2004. MMWR 2004;53:(No. SS-2).

[23] The US Preventive Task Force. Available at: www.ed.gov/policy/gen/guide. Accessed June 10, 2005.
     Family Educational Rights and Privacy Act (FERPA). Available at: www.uspreventivetaskforce.gov. Accessed May 15, 2005.

[24] US Department of Education. Available at: www.ed.gov/policy/gen/guid/fpco/ferpa/index.html. Accessed May 18, 2005.

[25] Health Insurance Portability and Accountability Act of 1996 (HIPPA). Available at: www.hhs.gov/ocr/privacy. Accessed June 12, 2005.

[26] National Institutes of Health, Office of Human Subjects Research. Guidelines for the conduct of research involving human subjects. 5th edition. Available at: http://ohsr.od.nih.gov/. Accessed June 9, 2005.

Nurs Clin N Am 40 (2005) 725–727

NURSING CLINICS
OF NORTH AMERICA

PREFACE

Nurse-Managed Health Centers

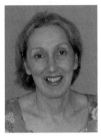

Barbara Rideout, MSN, APRN, BC

Guest Editor

F or more than a century nurses have been at the forefront of providing
health care to populations with limited access to care and of addressing
unmet health care needs of communities. When health care needs are unmet, somewhere a nurse rises to the occasion and takes care of it. Such names
as Florence Nightingale, Lillian Wald, and Margaret Sanger remind nurses of
our roots in the community and in the care of underserved populations. Hang-
ing on the wall of my office is a quote, given to me by a dear colleague as we
embarked on the opening of our first nurse-managed health center (NMHC):
"I look forward to the day when there are no nurses to the sick but only nurses
to the well," Florence Nightingale, 1893. It drives a personal practice philosophy that provides professional rewards each day when I leave our NMHC
knowing that I have made a difference in the health of at least one client.

Despite the wealth that exists in the United States, disparity in health exists
with regard to socioeconomic status. Health care is big business and is not
a "right" of each individual. This disparity exists across the lifespan, but it
is particularly evident for the working poor: men who are considered able-
bodied, who work every day, but at jobs that offer no access to health insurance and barely enough money to care for their family's basic needs; women
who as head of households lead lives so chaotic that they often are forced to
chose between coming for health care or providing food on the table for dinner;
and countless other disenfranchised groups.

0029-6465/05/$ – see front matter
doi:10.1016/j.cnur.2005.08.002

As this issue of *Nursing Clinics of North America* began to take shape, the recurring themes regardless of topic included health disparities, underserved populations, financial self-sufficiency for NMHCs, and the invisibility of NMHCs as true safety net providers. Today's visionary nurses, just as their well-known predecessors, are in an excellent position to provide high-quality health care that is accessible, cost-effective, and satisfying to clients. In many cases our patients receive access to more comprehensive services than their wealthier counterparts because they are cared for by advanced practice nurses who, by their education, approach care from a holistic perspective.

This issue of *Nursing Clinics of North America* presents the broad spectrum of health issues addressed by NMHCs in the United States. Perspectives are introduced related to decreasing health disparities by recognizing the work of NMHCs as true safety net providers and providing them with the much needed compensation that is provided to other federally funded providers. Hansen-Turton promotes the agenda for policy and advocacy of the National Nursing Centers Consortium that would recognize NMHCs as viable partners with the federal government to decrease health disparities. Campbell promotes a model for sustaining nurse-managed practices by identifying nursing as the practice, articulating a practice mission, and creating a team approach. Anderko and coworkers encourage the formation of practice-based research networks to define relevant research questions and acceptable methods in partnership with the community to translate research into practice, improve health outcomes, and ultimately change health policy based on the evidence. Beidler encourages the use of an ethical framework to anticipate and address the distress that occurs in providers while advocating for patients through and around existing barriers to health care access.

From the grass roots perspective we look at a smattering of "best practices" gleaned from across the United States. Ferrari and Rideout promote the marriage of public health nursing and primary care by advanced practice nurses in providing a mutually supportive approach to health care of a poor urban community in one of the largest cities in the country. McDevitt and coworkers discuss their model of integrating primary and mental health care for persons with serious and persistent mental illness. Youssey and colleagues demonstrate the use of Healthy People 2010 objectives to provide for urgent and chronic health care of homeless children. Dawley and Beam examine the historical perspective of nurses visiting with pregnant women and describe a reincarnation of the Olds model to provide services to pregnant women and their children through the Nurse Family Partnership. Plowfield and coworkers describe their use of the OMAHA documentation system to capture health promotion, education, and disease prevention outreach services to the well elderly.

This issue can only begin to scratch the surface of all the wonderful programs being offered by nurses. It focuses on the many issues that face nurses whose labor of love is to provide high-quality care that is accessible, cost-effective, culturally sensitive, and satisfactory to the most vulnerable populations.

I look forward to the day when every citizen, regardless of status and ability to pay, has the option of choosing to receive health care at a NMHC.

Barbara Rideout, MSN, APRN, BC
Drexel University College of Nursing and Health Professions
1505 Race Street
Mail Stop 501
Philadelphia, PA 19102, USA

E-mail address: bwr23@drexel.edu

Nurs Clin N Am 40 (2005) 729–738

NURSING CLINICS
OF NORTH AMERICA

ELSEVIER
SAUNDERS

The Nurse-Managed Health Center Safety Net: a Policy Solution to Reducing Health Disparities

Tine Hansen-Turton, MGA

National Nursing Centers Consortium, 260 South Broad Street, 18th Floor, Philadelphia, PA 19102, USA

The United States health care system has become increasingly complex. Safety net providers deliver a significant level of health care to the un- and underinsured and other vulnerable populations. With more than 40 million Americans without health insurance, countless undocumented immigrants, increases in health care spending, and cuts in Medicaid funding, this safety net is more essential than ever [1]. New and innovative approaches to the health care system and the safety net are needed to maximize the quality of care, improve accessibility, increase cost-effectiveness, and fulfill patient expectations. Through the establishment of nurse-managed health centers (NMHCs), certified registered nurse practitioners (CRNPs) and other advanced practice nurses have created a safety net that meet these goals and the demands of the vulnerable populations they serve.

THE SAFETY NET

In a 2000 report summarizing America's safety net, the Institute of Medicine (IOM) found that the health care safety net is neither secure nor uniform in its ability to provide adequate health care coverage to vulnerable populations. It attributes this variation to the number of uninsured in the local health care market, the coverage of federal and state programs such as Medicaid, and the general political and economic environment. The report further noted that a consistent definition of the health care safety net has not been developed [2]. The core safety net providers as listed in the IOM summary are

Some data used to support the Findings and Policy Implications come from an evaluation sponsored by the Centers for Medicare and Medicaid Services, entitled The Nursing Center Model of Health Care for the Underserved. The statements contained in The Nursing Center Model of Health care for the Underserved report are solely those of the authors and do not necessarily reflect the views or policies of the Health Care Financing Administration.

E-mail address: tine@nncc.us

community health centers (CHCs), federally qualified health centers (FQHCs), public hospitals, and local health departments. Also discussed are other providers, who may not receive federal funding targeted to safety net providers, but nevertheless provide care to underserved populations. These include community and teaching hospitals, private practitioners, private rural and urban physicians, school-based health centers, the Veteran Health Administration, and the Indian Health Service [2]. Missing from this list are NMHCs, despite their long history of providing low-income, medically underserved, vulnerable populations with accessible, culturally acceptable, and affordable primary care and health promotion services. This omission led to a federally funded evaluation of NMHCs for recognition as safety net providers, results of which will be detailed further in this article.

THE NURSE-MANAGED HEALTH CENTERS

NMHCs are managed by nurses in partnership with the communities that they serve [3]. They usually are located in medically underserved areas in urban and rural communities and represent a growing movement of health centers that appear to be a critical but hidden safety net. They reduce health disparities by providing accessible comprehensive primary care and community health programs aimed at health promotion and disease prevention, in addition to behavioral health and home-care services [3]. NMHCs focus care on patients, their families, and their communities. Serving medically underserved urban and rural areas, many NMHCs operate in areas suffering from health profession shortages, providing care to low-income, minority, homeless, and migrant families. Their physical locations include public housing developments, schools, churches, community centers, and shelters. In NMHCs, health problems and potential health problems are not viewed in isolation, but within the context of societal, environmental, and cultural influences that have impacted the patient's past and present health and that have the potential to impact future health. Patients are connected with resources that address and correct the forces that have impacted their health negatively. Providers within nurse-managed centers view their patients as partners in care and provide patients with the knowledge and skills to empower them so that they can assume responsibility for their own health, make informed decisions about their health, and become their own advocates. Care is provided by CRNPs serving as primary care providers, clinical nurse specialists, nurse midwives, registered nurses, health educators, community outreach workers, and collaborating physicians, providing medical back up and consultation. CRNPs are experts at disease prevention and health promotion and are certified to diagnose and manage illness. A *Journal of the American Medical Association* study of 1316 primary care patients, randomly assigned to either CRNPs or physicians, strongly supported that delivery of primary care between the two providers did not differ and found patient outcomes comparable in the two groups [4].

Over 250 NMHCs operate throughout the United States. Although today's NMHCs trace their immediate roots to changes in national health care laws initiated in the mid-1960s, the nursing model of holistic care that integrates health promotion with primary care and focuses on serving vulnerable populations dates back to the late nineteenth century. In the 1890s, social activists such as Lillian Wald, founder of the Henry Street Settlement, and Margaret Sanger, founder of the first birth control clinic in New York, introduced the earliest nursing models of service. Since the late 1970s, in conjunction with the development of educational programs for CRNPs through funding from the Health Resources and Services Administration's (HRSA) Division of Nursing, faculties in schools of nursing have established NMHCs. In addition to providing necessary services to the community, these linkages have provided clinical sites for educating nurses at all levels and settings for faculty practice. Although academic-based NMHCs are a common model, there are also hospital-based and freestanding community-based centers. All of them provide patients with accessible, affordable, and quality health care.

A 2003 to 2004 national survey of member centers conducted by the National Nursing Centers Consortium (NNCC) showed that the centers serve 64% racial and ethnic minority populations (African American, Latino, Asian, and others). Sixty-three percent of the patients are under the age of 35, and up to 50% of the patients are uninsured. Findings have also shown the CRNPs are cost-effective [5]. NMHCs cut health care costs, because by treating the uninsured, they reduce emergency room usage and thereby save Medicaid costs. The average primary care encounter cost for clients treated by NMHCs participating in the CHC program is 10% less then the primary care encounter cost for CHCs managed by physicians. The average personnel cost for NMHCs participating in the CHC program is 11% less than the personnel costs for CHCs managed by physicians [6]. Geriatric health promotion and disease prevention programs run by NMHCs help cut annual health care costs by as much as $ 37,500,000 [7].

THE NATIONAL NURSING CENTERS CONSORTIUM

Despite the effectiveness of NMHCs, they work under the radar of the general public and thus have not received the same level of visibility as CHCs and other safety net providers as evidenced by the omission in the IOM report. Consequently, they rely on a patchwork of funding and struggle financially. To address the challenge of visibility and sustainability, nurse-managed health center leaders in the Philadelphia region partnered to form the Regional Nursing Centers Consortium as an umbrella organization and advocate for NMHCs. This idea quickly caught on to others, and since its inception as an informal association in 1996, hiring its first staff in the summer of 1998, the Consortium became NNCC, a 501(c) [2] nonprofit, in 2002. NNCC now serves over 150 NMHCs, providing care to over 1.5 million people across America [3]. The NNCC's mission is to strengthen the capacity, growth, and development of NMHCs to provide quality health care services to vulnerable populations and to eliminate health disparities in underserved communities. Its main focus is to make NMHCs sustainable through policy and advocacy efforts at the state and federal levels. The NNCC provides its member NMHCs with services designed to assist them in meeting challenges they face in today's rapidly moving health care environment. This involves facilitating the sharing of best practices among NMHCs nationally and providing comprehensive technical assistance and fundraising support to its member centers.

NNCC has an ambitious policy and advocacy agenda. Since its inception, the NNCC has been instrumental in assisting national members in receiving prescriptive authority at state levels, having CRNPs and advanced practice nurses defined as primary care providers, and raising over $30 million dollars to date, from local, state, and federal contracts and grants, Congressional appropriations, and private foundations. It also has educated third party payers, such as health insurance plans, which has resulted in some health plans changing their policies to include CRNPs and NMHCs in both their Medicaid/Medicare and private insurance products. A major push has been to get NMHCs either FQHC or CHC designation and prospective payment. This past year, the US Senate Report 108-345 included several supporting policy requests, such as urging the Agency for Health care Research and Quality and the National Institutes of Nursing Research to include and increase funding for NMHCs and advanced practice nurses in research and demonstration projects [8]. Congress also recognized that NMHCs serve a dual function in strengthening the health care safety net by providing health care to populations in underserved areas and by providing the clinical experiences to nursing students that are mandatory for professional development. Recognizing that NMHCs are frequently the only source of health care to their patients and that a lack of clinical education sites for nurses is a contributing factor to the nationwide nursing shortage, the committee encourages HRSA to provide alternative means to secure cost-based reimbursement for NMHCs, by providing that reimbursement or by granting university-based CHCs. In addition, the committee urges HRSA to research the effectiveness of NMHCs as a national model to reduce health disparities [8].

Finally, the US Senate encouraged the Administration on Aging to facilitate demonstration projects of nurse-managed geriatric wellness centers [8].

CHALLENGES TO THE NURSE-MANAGED MODEL OF CARE

The contributions of NMHCs to the core safety net have been made in relative anonymity, partly because of a dearth of literature outside of the nursing profession documenting the services that they provide to medically underserved, vulnerable populations [9]. As a result of working under the radar, they were excluded from the IOM's list of providers that comprise America's health care safety net.

NMHCs face the same obstacles as other safety net providers. The comprehensive primary care and enabling services offered by safety net providers rarely generate enough funds to cover their costs [2]. This is particularly the case for most NMHCs, as they are not CHCs or FQHCs and are unable to receive cost-based reimbursement, now called prospective payment [10]. By receiving cost-based reimbursement like federally funded community health centers, NMHCs would be in a position to offset the cost of caring for the uninsured, because they will receive a higher level of reimbursement for Medicaid and Medicare patients. For core safety net providers that fall under Section 330 of the Public Health Service Act, Medicaid compensation programs have narrowed the gap between the providers' expenses and their revenues [2]. Many NMHCs are not eligible for these compensation programs and must rely on multiple, and often inconsistent, funding streams. Those who have the most difficulty receiving CHC or FQHC status tend to be the academic NMHCs in private universities.

NATIONAL NURSING CENTERS CONSORTIUM'S RESPONSE TO CHALLENGES

To address the dearth of data and literature describing the full scope of services provided by NMHCs, and ultimately to increase awareness and ensure sustainability of NMHCs, the 2002 budget appropriation language for the Centers for Medicare and Medicaid Services (CMS) [11] and the accompanying conference committee report included the statement for the NNCC to initiate a demonstration project to evaluate NMHCs in urban and rural areas across Pennsylvania, the state with the most centers. In response to the Senate language, the NNCC wrote a proposal to CMS, which had the following two objectives:

- To create an extensive descriptive evaluation of clients served and services provided at primary care NMHCs in Pennsylvania
- To compare select population-based measures of quality and health care resource use of NMHCs with those of like providers including community health centers

As the national organization of NMHCs, the NNCC was positioned uniquely to conduct this demonstration project. It also previously had established a practice-based research network linking several of its member health centers through a common database, which gave the centers the capability to conduct an evaluation. The 2004 report to the CMS, entitled *The Nursing Model of Health care for the Underserved,* answers a specific challenge; it provides documentation of the ability of NMHCs to serve as core safety net providers in America's health care system. It showed that NMHCs meet the IOM's definition of safety net provider and address health disparities with culturally sensitive and cost-efficient care [12].

REDUCING HEALTH DISPARITIES: FINDINGS FROM THE CENTERS FOR MEDICARE AND MEDICAID SERVICES EVALUATION

The CMS report found that consistent with their mission to offer care to patients regardless of their ability to pay, NMHCs give care to numerous uninsured clients with limited ability to pay for their care. Like IOM-defined safety net providers, NMHCs provide a full range of health care services, including primary care, behavioral health care, and preventive care such as health education and disease prevention. In fact, the evaluation found that, in comparison with like providers such as CHCs, NMHCs:

- Have higher rates of generic medication fills and lower rates of hospitalizations
- Are on par in the rate of emergency room visits
- Are on par in the use of appropriate medications for people with asthma
- Provide similar enabling services without the same level of funding

The report's findings are highlighted in this section.

Enabling services
Findings
All NMHCs provided health education and environmental health risk reduction; 89% provided outreach, transportation, interpretation and translation services, and eligibility assistance. Seventy-eight percent provided home visiting and case-management, and 67% provided parenting education. Other services include discharge planning, nursing home placement, and special education. Additionally, the health centers offer services such as summer camp, grand parenting education, food assistance, blood pressure and stroke screening, adolescent support groups, family planning, dentistry, podiatry, prenatal care, and fitness and nutrition programs.

Implications
NMHCs provide similar enabling services as CHCs/FQHCs without the same level of funding. In many instances they are providing expanded enabling services to meet the needs of their communities.

Patient satisfaction
Findings
Patients were surveyed using the Medical Outcomes Trust Patient Satisfaction tool. Analysis of questions pertaining to patient access to health care and manner of health care delivered to patients by their primary care providers showed mean aggregate scores, ranging from 4.03 to 4.19 on a five-point scale. A score of five indicates excellent, and a score of one indicates poor.

Implications
Findings suggest that patients were highly satisfied with the accessibility and delivery of care at NMHCs. This finding coincides with existing literature, which has shown that patients consistently have rated their satisfaction with care from CRNPs as high [13].

Health Plan Employer Data and Information Set measures and use rates
Findings
The comparison analysis focused on several specific Health Plan Employer Data and Information Set (HEDIS) measures and use measures. HEDIS measures provide consumers with information detailing the performance of health

care providers. For this study, measures appropriate to the safety net population were chosen. On the measures included, NMHCs had higher rates of generic medication fills and lower rates of hospitalizations than like providers, such as community health centers. In addition, NMHCs had a higher patient retention rate. NMHCs demonstrated parity in the rate of emergency room visits per 1000 members and use of appropriate medications for people with asthma. NMHCs had a lower annual prevalence of chlamydia screening.

Implications

These findings are an indicator of the quality of care provided by NMHCs. Their performance rate was very similar on key measures to other recognized safety net providers, such as CHCs and FQHCs.

Financial reimbursement

Findings

Thirty-seven percent of the health center revenues come from Medicaid-managed care plans, 23% from private foundations, 23% from government contracts and grants, 6% from private donors, 6% from Medicare, and 5% from private pay or other sources. Five of the participating NMHCs have been successful in receiving FQHC status. Of the five centers, four also have been successful in receiving community health center grant funds. As such, these five health centers receive a higher level of funding from the government and a lower level of funding from foundations than non-FQHCs. The remaining health centers, however, have a high dependence on private foundation funding for their uninsured and Medicaid managed care for their Medicaid patients.

Implications

The NMHCs that have been successful in competing for and qualifying for CHC/FQHC status are the most financially stable health centers and most able to continue to serve as a safety net providers.

Demographics

Findings

Demographic distinctions arise based on center location. In urban health centers, 87% of patients served are black. In the migrant health center, 99% of patients served are Hispanic. In the rural health center, nearly 100% of the patients served are white. Patients of the suburban health centers are the most racially and ethnically diverse, as 38% of the patients are black; 35% are Hispanic; 21% are white, and 5% are Asian. Patients in the rural nurse-managed health center are older, and males 45 to 64 years of age constitute the largest group. Urban, suburban, and migrant centers serve a large proportion of children and youth under the age of 20, 45% of their patient base. Twenty-five percent of patients are young adults, between 20 and 29 years of age. Overall, 61% of patients are female.

Implications

The findings show that the centers serve a diverse population through all age groups with a focus on children and youth, suggesting the centers are getting services to underserved populations at an early age critical to providing preventive health.

Insurance status
Findings

Of the patients seen at all NMHCs, 35% were uninsured; 40% received Medicaid; 17% had commercial health insurance, and 9% received Medicare benefits. In the migrant nurse-managed health center, 99% of the population served were uninsured.

Implications

The findings suggest that the centers meet the IOM's definition of safety net provider. Insurance status is an indicator of economic status and well-being. This confirms that a substantial share of the patient mix at NMHCs is uninsured or on Medicaid, demonstrating the vulnerability of the people served.

Employment status
Findings

Of the urban patients seen in NMHCs, 53% reported being employed; 33% reported being unemployed, and 14% reported being students.

Implications

NMHCs provide care to vulnerable populations. The findings suggest that the working poor are less likely to be insured. Lack of access to health care is an indicator of poor economic status.

Health disparities diagnoses and health services

The evaluation found that NMHCs serve a population impacted by health disparities and perform a broad range of diagnoses and procedures, many of which address health disparities directly.

Findings

Preventive health constituted the largest diagnostic category, followed by reproductive health and behavioral health. Among urban, suburban, and migrant centers, analysis revealed behavioral health to be the most frequent health disparity diagnosis, followed by hypertension, diabetes, asthma, and obesity. Asthma-related diagnoses represented 32% of all pulmonary diagnoses; hypertension represented 77% of all cardiovascular diagnoses. Diabetes and obesity represented 69% and 25% of all metabolic diagnoses, respectively. At the rural center, the top three diagnoses were respiratory-related, hypertension, and diabetes. Disparity diagnoses such as hypertension, diabetes, depression, asthma, and obesity were among the top 15 diagnoses overall.

Implications

The findings suggest that NMHCs directly address health disparities. Preventive health, such as immunizations, screenings, and health education, is the focal point in their care delivery. Preventive health also is considered one of the most critical factors in eliminating health disparities. Further, the centers integrate behavioral health with primary care services, another critical factor in eliminating health disparities.

POLICY CONSIDERATIONS FOR THE HEALTH CARE COMMUNITY AND LOOKING TO THE FUTURE

Nurse-managed health centers are safety net providers

Like IOM-defined safety net providers, the CMS-sponsored evaluation found that NMHCs deliver a significant level of health care to the uninsured, patients who are on Medicaid, and other vulnerable patients. Consistent with their mission to offer care to patients regardless of their ability to pay, NMHCs give care to numerous uninsured clients with limited ability to pay for their care. NMHCs are clearly safety net providers.

Nurse-managed health centers provide a medical home for the underserved

Like IOM-defined safety net providers, NMHCs provide a full range of health care services, including primary care, preventive care, and behavioral health care to the uninsured, patients who are on Medicaid, and other vulnerable patients.

Nurse-managed medical centers struggle financially and need cost-based reimbursement to be sustainable

The major obstacle NMHCs face is the struggle for financial sustainability. The comprehensive primary care and enabling services offered by these providers rarely generate enough funds to cover their costs. Furthermore, the unique payer and patient mix of NMHCs, which includes numerous uninsured and Medicaid patients, precludes the flexibility to shift costs. In contrast, CHCs, which receive cost-based reimbursement for Medicaid and Medicare patients, in addition to grant funds to serve uninsured, have a greater ability to sustain operations. Thus, NMHCs need cost-based reimbursement to be sustainable.

Nurse-managed health centers should be recognized as safety net providers and are viable partners with the federal government to reduce health disparities

The data demonstrate that NMHCs are instrumental in addressing and eliminating health disparities, and that they should be recognized formally as core safety net providers, equivalent to CHCs. Currently, the government underuses NMHCs as safety net providers. Given federal recognition, NMHCs could achieve financial parity with like providers, allowing them to serve as a sustainable safety net. Thus, NMHCs are in a unique position to be a partner with the federal government to increase access health care services and to reduce health disparities.

In conclusion, regardless of the promise that NMHCs hold as safety net providers, their future continues to be threatened. With soaring health care costs at the state and federal levels and severe cuts in Medicaid, all non-CHC safety net providers are at risk. Without proper government and foundation support from funders, the ultimate result could be that un- and underinsured consumers will have no providers to turn to for their care. America then would face a health care crisis, and no health disparities would be addressed.

Acknowledgements

The author wishes to acknowledge the assistance of NNCC's Project Associate and Policy Analyst, Michelle O'Connell, MGA, in the preparation of this manuscript.

References

[1] Levit K, Smith C, Cowan C, et al. Inflation spurs health spending in 2000. Health Aff 2002;21(1):172–81.

[2] Institute of Medicine. Summary: America's healthcare safety net, intact but endangered. Washington, DC: National Academics press; 2000.

[3] Coleman S, Hansen-Turton T. Going national: National Nursing Centers Consortium. Advance for Nurses 2003;5(11):14–8.

[4] Mundinger MO, Kane RL, Totten AM, et al. Primary outcomes in patients treated by nurse practitioners or physicians. JAMA 2000;88:59–68.

[5] Venning P, et al. Randomised controlled trial comparing cost effectiveness of general practitioners and nurse practitioners in primary care. BMJ 2000;320:1048–53.

[6] Leiyu S. 1996–2001 Uniform Data System (UDS) for health centers with 330 funding: Bureau of Primary Health Care.

[7] Lorig KR. Evidence suggesting that a chronic disease self-management program can improve health status while reducing hospitalization: a randomized control trial. Med Care 1999;37(1):5–14.

[8] S. REP. NO. 108-345 at 37 (2005).

[9] Anderko L, Kinton E. Speaking with a unified voice: recommendations for the collection of aggregated outcome data in nurse-managed centers. Policy, Politics and Nursing Practice 2001;(4):295–303.

[10] Hansen-Turton T, Kinsey K. The quest for self-sustainability: nurse-managed health centers meeting the policy challenge. Policy, Politics and Nursing Practice 2001;2(4):304–9.

[11] Department of Health and Human Services Appropriations Act. 2002. Pub L. No 107–116, § 9921, 115 Stat. 2177, 2193.

[12] Hansen-Turton T, Line L, O'Connell M, et al. The nursing center model of healthcare for the underserved. HCFA Contract No. 18–P91720/3–01.

[13] Uppal S, Lee C, Mielcarek M, et al. A comparison of patient satisfaction with conventional and nurse led outpatient follow-up after grommet insertion. Auris Nasus Larynx 2004;31: 23–8.

Nurs Clin N Am 40 (2005) 739–745

NURSING CLINICS
OF NORTH AMERICA

Sustaining Nurse-Managed Practice

Linda Campbell, PhD, RN

Loretto Heights Department of Nursing, Rueckert-Hartman School for Health Professions,
Regis University, 3333 Regis Boulevard, G-8, Denver, CO 80221, USA

C ommunity-based nurse-managed practice (CBNMP) offers local populations the opportunity to contract directly with professional nurses for primary health care services [1]. Despite provision of high quality care below the average cost of primary care providers [2–7], a 21% decline in the number of known academic CBNMPs was calculated between 1989 and 1998 [5,8]. Closure of these CBNMPs resulted in a loss of cost-effective primary health care for their vulnerable service populations, and disrupted clinical practitioner education programs and programs of research. Anecdotal evidence suggests similar declines for nurse-managed practices in nonacademic settings [9].

METHODS

An institutional review board-approved multiple case study was conducted from 2002 to 2003 at CBNMPs in prevalent practice contexts: urban-academic, urban-private/not-for-profit, and rural-federally qualified health centers. The three sites were located within a 50-mile radius in a state in the south central part of the United States. The study addressed factors believed to facilitate or hinder the innovation development process of CBNMP.

A model synthesizing concepts from Diffusion of Innovations [10] and Community as Partner [11] was used to construct 20 variables of interest. Data collection on those variables proceeded through four strategies: background survey, document review, observations, and interviews (N = 85). Rigorously conducted procedures included 29 days of data collection during two site visits totaling 9 or 10 days at each site. Thematic and matrix analyses facilitated triangulation of qualitative and quantitative findings.

This work was supported by grant number 5 F31 NR07573-02 from the National Institutes of Health/National Institute for Nursing Research, with additional funding from Sigma Theta Tau International (Alpha Kappa chapter-at-large) and the Nursing Economics Foundation.

E-mail address: lcampbel@regis.edu

0029-6465/05/$ – see front matter
doi:10.1016/j.cnur.2005.08.007

RESULTS

The study described and compared the evolution of the innovation development process for CBNMPs in three practice settings. Narrative profiles were compiled for each site, and then commonalties across sites were identified. Commonalties included diminished reliance on grant or federal funding, increased size of practice, increased diversity and acuity among patients, and transformation from local clinic to citywide or regional practice (Box 1).

To highlight a few of the factors, a mix of communication channels included diffusion by word of mouth and community partnerships. Champions of CBNMP included community members, like a mayor's wife and local clergy, and funding sources, like the Kellogg Foundation or a school of nursing. Becoming embedded in a community occurred through years of service or community development activities, wisely required by initial grant funding. Factors that hindered diffusion and sustainability of CBNMP included:

- Insufficiently planned transition from grant funding
- Resistance or invisibility within the community
- Lack of referral sources
- Abrupt change in payer or service population
- Inadequate reimbursements
- Laggards
- Turnover of advanced practice nurses

Most of the hindering factors are self-explanatory, but laggards warrant further explanation. Laggards included potential patients who had never come to a CBNMP. At one site, an informant said, "They may not be educated. They may not care. They may have a drug problem or a mental health problem. They may have obligations in their family. They may be undocumented workers." At all sites, potential patients typically had not heard about the CBNMP

Box 1: Factors found to facilitate diffusion and sustainability of the community-based nurse-managed practice

Supportive infrastructure

Adherence to the sponsoring organization's mission

Full-time delivery of primary health care by advanced practice nurses

Services based on periodic community assessments

A mix of communication channels

Growth from a steady stream of diverse users

A mix of payers

Collaboration and referral with other health care providers

Champions of CBNMP

Becoming embedded in the community

or held misconceptions. For example, one community informant thought nurse-managed practice was "inner city stuff for people who can't afford a doctor."

Of note, grant funding and autonomy simultaneously facilitated and hindered diffusion and sustainability of CBNMPs. Specifically, grant funding that facilitated development at the urban sites also provoked tension among advanced practice nurses and administrators because of grant requirements for simultaneous community development. In particular, many advanced practice nurses resented limited resources being used to convene focus groups and develop community partnerships. In addition, grant funding typically was limited to one or two cycles, which required skill sets and business acumen not included in most advanced practice nurses' education. Moreover, autonomous primary health care could pose a competitive threat when the CBNMPs were seen as a choice for health care, ironically, even when other providers did not accept the CBNMPs' service populations or insurance plans.

DISCUSSION

All study sites demonstrated sustainability through impressive adoption statistics and solid evidence of being embedded in their communities. Factors identified as critical to sustainability focused on adequate reimbursement and continued provision of primary health care services. Unequivocally, the literature cited reimbursement for services as the critical factor for sustainability across all types of CBNMP [3,9,12]. In addition, Mundinger [6] made an eloquent plea for fee equity with physicians. For many centers, however, so many patients are either uninsured or so poorly insured that adequate revenue cannot be realized for their services [9,13].

Study sites identified other factors for sustainability as well, including more acceptance of advanced practice nursing and continued patient satisfaction, which approximated recommendations in the literature [14,15]. Of note, turnover among providers, while undesirable, was survivable at study sites. In fact, as predicted by Rogers' theory [10], most innovators had moved on to other endeavors. For example, one site's nurse practitioner manager exemplified innovator behavior by moving on after a 5-year period at each of two previous sites. Her current role as nurse practitioner manager, however, permitted a satisfying combination of two favorite endeavors, seeing patients and having more avenues for innovation. She successfully had developed a second CBNMP in a mostly Hispanic community and planned a third CBNMP to serve the area's burgeoning population of uninsured refugees.

Simultaneous help and hindrance of some factors were corroborated by one qualitative study and attributed to the complexities associated with CBNMPs [12]. For example, although grants may launch a CBNMP or enable provision of needs-targeted services, they do not enhance the margin or long-term sustainability of CBNMPs by themselves. A mix of payers, which may include foundations that award grants, are needed for sustainable CBNMPs.

Finally, study sites did not mention nursing research among factors for sustainability, as recommended in the literature [14,16]. They reported user data to their sponsoring organizations but did not have well-developed programs of research. Barriers to conducting research included lack of time and lack of access to an on-site management information system, which mirrored obstacles noted in the literature [17,18]. Lack of a nursing theoretical framework also may affect a CBNMP's impetus to engage in research [19].

Future research is expected to refine the innovation development process of CBNMPs and eventually permit a stronger, unified voice for CBNMPs that communicates their cost-effective, high quality outcomes. In this way, CBNMPs will fulfill their promise to be "nursing's quintessential contribution to 21st Century health care" [19].

RECOMMENDATIONS

CBNMPs need to look within and without the nursing profession for principles that promote authentic, self-sustaining practice. Within nursing, sustainable academic CBNMPs may depend on the willingness of a sponsoring academic institution to provide services that may not be self-supporting [7]. For example, faculty-based practice offers a unique teaching function, which could be viewed as an in-kind return on investment. The National Organization of Nurse Practitioner Faculties has national linkages and on-line resource centers to support community health and faculty practice (www.nonpf.com).

In addition, research must document the processes and outcomes of sustainable CBNMP. Since completion of the study described in this article, the Michigan Academic Consortium has concluded a major Kellogg-funded grant. Their endeavor is replete with results of research on financial matters, outcomes, personnel issues, nurse practitioner education, and patient satisfaction (http://www.nnnmhc.org/eduResources.htm). Moreover, the consortium has evolved into the National Network of Nurse Managed Health Centers (http://www.nnnmhc.org), which held a national data consensus conference in December 2004. A final report documents progress made toward a minimum data set for CBNMP (http://www.nnnmhc.org/reports.htm).

Beyond the nursing profession, two business resources offer guidance for sustainable CBNMP: Built to Last: Successful Habits of Visionary Companies [20] and The Circle of Innovation [21]. Their counsel suggests ways to frame findings from this study and existing literature. Specifically, CBNMPs must proclaim their compelling distinction in primary health care delivery through the following seven imperatives.

First, CBNMPs must articulate a mission in support of exemplary practice, because an organizational vision is more important than a charismatic leader or particular product [20]. Then CBNMPs must seek interdisciplinary collaboration with business and public affairs professionals to determine if the mission of a potential infrastructure would support autonomous practice. CBNMPs also might consider developing a practice with nonacademic sponsors, such as private hospital charitable foundations.

Second, CBNMPs must identify their practice as nursing, operate from nursing theoretical frameworks that communicate nursing's holistic approach, and contribute to nursing science [19]. Then, CBNMPs must develop a set of core values that flow from the nursing theoretical framework. In particular, CBNMPs must embrace core values that allow for passionate pursuit of primary health care delivery and acceptance of tension and paradoxical situations [21]. The phrase "genius of the AND" [20] describes coexisting contradictory forces; an exemplary CBNMP will align with a core ideology and adapt to its environment.

Third, CBNMPs must create a professional team approach to support exemplary practice. CBNMPs delivering the full scope of primary health care services need various contributions with differing expertise from volunteers, nursing and business students, support staff, advanced practice nurses, administrators, and community champions. Staff members, regardless of role, should have a professional, problem-solving approach. They should be hired for intelligence, attitude, and diversity and be educated for needed skill sets [21]. Permitting various staff members to remain within their center of expertise while nurturing new skills may enhance their retention.

Champions of CBNMP may emerge from creation of extensive networks with sponsoring organizations, with press outlets, in service on community boards, and through position papers and other reports to governmental agencies. In particular, communication with the public through media advocacy may help to articulate the effectiveness of CBNMP [22–24].

Fourth, CBNMPs must balance mission with margin. Although initial grant funding may permit margin before mission, a CBNMP must plan from the beginning to balance its mission with fiscally responsible management. CBNMPs must reconsider their singular alignment with one service population, which may provoke insurmountable challenges in the face of abrupt change, especially in payers. Although it is admirable, rewarding, and vitally important to serve populations that would not receive care otherwise, CBNMPs must weigh the implications of serving only underprivileged populations and contemplate ways to subsidize indigent practices, rather than depend on them for fiscal sustainability. For example, a network of CBNMPs may bring holistic primary health care to an entire region, not just an isolated and impoverished community. In addition, CBNMPs must consider that anyone would want holistic primary health care delivered by a trusted advanced practice nurse who listens and cares about improving the health of individuals, families, and communities.

Fifth, CBNMPs must promote a "beautiful systems initiative" [21] and "say yes to wow" [21] to promote attractive practice sites that help develop a steady stream of diverse users. Only a population with no other option for health care would accept the sometimes decrepit conditions in which many CBNMPs initially locate their practice. CBNMPs must address their chronic invisibility not through market research but through educating and communicating with potential patients and payers. Then CBNMPs might package advanced practice nursing services differently so that potential populations would consider paying out-of-pocket, as they do for beauty treatments and complementary care providers.

Sixth, CBNMPs need to plan not only for growth but also for different types of leadership during the innovation development process. One leader may be superior at initiation; another leader may excel during social system integration. In fact, CBNMPs may need to draw their mentors from generations of leaders with varying skills, including faculty administrators and instructors, agency leadership, experienced nurse practitioners, and physicians. Semiretired physicians at two of the study's sites found a mutually beneficial arrangement, and they were held in high esteem. Semiretired nurses and nursing faculty may wish to extend their careers in a similar fashion.

CBNMPs could benefit immediately by expanding their definition of mentors. For example, the literature is replete with lessons learned in the development of CBNMPs [6,7,12,17,25]. In addition, since 2002, the National Nursing Centers Consortium has sponsored an annual conference of member centers. Its mission is to strengthen the capacity, growth, and development of nurse-managed health centers to provide quality health care services to vulnerable populations and eliminate health disparities in underserved communities (http://www.nationalnursingcenters.org).

Finally, CBNMPs must apply for local and national awards to increase their visibility and their professional and political clout. Faculty managers of CBNMPs might apply for university awards or alumni awards; city-wide CBNMPs might seek mayor's awards; regional CBNMPs might qualify for awards from state nursing associations, and influential leaders might garner awards from Sigma Theta Tau International or nursing journals.

SUMMARY

A multiple case study of CBNMPs in prevalent practice contexts revealed factors that facilitated or hindered the innovation development process of CBNMPs. Critical facilitating factors included a supportive infrastructure, full-time delivery of needs-driven primary health care by advanced practice nurses, and growth from a steady stream of diverse users and a mix of payers. Noteworthy hindering factors included insufficiently planned transition from initial grant funding, invisibility of the CBNMP within the community, lack of referral sources, and inadequate reimbursements. To promote sustainable practice, CBNMPs should articulate a practice mission, identify the practice as nursing, create a team approach, balance mission with margin, and promote attractive practice sites. Other recommendations include planning for growth and evolution of health care and applying for awards to increase the visibility and political clout of CBNMPs.

References

[1] Holman EJ. Council update. Nurs Health Care 1992;13(5):261.
[2] Burgener SC, Moore SJ. The role of advanced practice nurses in community settings. Nurs Econ 2002;20(3):102–8.

[3] Hansen-Turton T, Kinsey K. The quest for self-sustainability: nurse-managed health centers meeting the policy challenge. Policy, Politics & Nursing Practice 2001;2(4):304–9.

[4] Helvie CO. Efficacy of primary care in a nursing center. Nurs Case Manag 1999;4(4): 201–16.

[5] Matherlee K. The nursing center in concept and practice (issue brief 746). In: Matherlee K, editor. Proceedings of the National Health Policy Forum. Washington (DC): George Washington University; 1999. p. 1–10.

[6] Mundinger MO. Can advanced practice nurses succeed in the primary care market? Nurs Econ 1999;17(1):7–14.

[7] Spitzer R. The Vanderbilt University experience. Nurs Manage 1997;28(3):38–40.

[8] Aydelotte MK, Gregory MS. Nursing practice: innovative models. In: Nursing centers: meeting the demand for quality health care (Pub No 21–2311). New York: National League for Nursing; 1989. p. 1–20.

[9] Lockhart CA. Community nursing centers: an analysis of status and needs. In: Murphy B, editor. Nursing centers: the time is now. New York: National League for Nursing; 1995. p. 1–18.

[10] Rogers EM. Diffusion of innovations. 4th edition. New York: The Free Press; 1995.

[11] Anderson ET, McFarlane J. Community as partner: theory and practice in nursing. 3rd edition. Philadelphia: Lippincott; 2000.

[12] Seamon J, Oakley D, Pohl J, et al. Academic nurse-managed centers: what does it take to succeed? Mich Nurse 2000;11:12–3.

[13] Anderko L, Uscian M. Quality outcome measures at an academic rural nurse-managed center: a core safety net provider. Policy, Politics & Nursing Practice 2001;2(4):288–94.

[14] Phillips DL, Steel JE. Factors influencing scope of practice in nursing centers. J Prof Nurs 1994;10(2):84–90.

[15] Nash MG, Blackwood D, Boone EB, et al. Managing expectations between patient and nurse. J Nurs Adm 1994;24(11):49–55.

[16] Walker PH. A comprehensive community nursing center model: maximizing practice income—a challenge to educators. J Prof Nurs 1994;10(3):131–9.

[17] Oros M, Johantgen M, Antol S, et al. Community-based nursing centers: challenges and opportunities in implementation and sustainability. Policy, Politics & Nursing Practice 2001; 2(4):277–87.

[18] Barger SE. Establishing a nursing center: learning from the literature and the experiences of others. J Prof Nurs 1995;11(4):203–12.

[19] Barrett EAM. Nursing centers without nursing frameworks: what's wrong with this picture? Nurs Sci Q 1993;6(3):115–7.

[20] Collins JC, Porras JI. Built to last: successful habits of visionary companies. 2nd edition. New York: Harper Business; 1994.

[21] Peters T. The circle of innovation. New York: Vintage; 1997.

[22] Norwood SL. The invisibility of advanced practice nurses in popular magazines. J Am Acad Nurs Pract 2001;13(3):129–33.

[23] Chaffee M. Health communications: nursing education for increased visibility and effectiveness. J Prof Nurs 2000;16(1):31–8.

[24] Flynn BC. Communicating with the public: community-based nursing research and practice. Public Health Nurs 1998;15(3):165–70.

[25] Zachariah R, Lundeen SP. Research and practice in an academic community nursing center. Image: The Journal of Nursing Scholarship 1997;29(3):255–60.

Nurs Clin N Am 40 (2005) 747–758

NURSING CLINICS
OF NORTH AMERICA

ELSEVIER
SAUNDERS

Practice-Based Research Networks: Nursing Centers and Communities Working Collaboratively to Reduce Health Disparities

Laura Anderko, RN, PhD*, Claudia Bartz, RN, PhD, FAAN, Sally Lundeen, RN, PhD, FAAN

College of Nursing, University of Wisconsin-Milwaukee, 1921 E. Hartford Avenue, Milwaukee, WI 53211, USA

As communities struggle to address the persistent problem of disparities in the use of health care and health outcomes for at-risk populations, the development of best practices for conducting research that translates into real-world situations has received increased attention. The populations most at risk are those disenfranchised from the mainstream health care system who have been historically distrustful of this system and its health care providers. Research methods and designs that capture the unique characteristics of these at-risk populations and the communities in which they live are particularly challenging to implement but critical to learning about these populations and developing effective intervention strategies.

One strategy for overcoming some of these barriers and improving the translation of conventional research methods into community settings is community-based participatory research (CBPR). CBPR is a collaborative approach to research that combines methods of inquiry with community capacity building strategies to bridge the gap between knowledge produced through research and what is practiced in communities to improve health. Interest is growing for academic institutions, health agencies, and communities to form CBPR partnerships, although few guidelines have established what resources are required to promote successful collaborative research efforts [1].

Another strategy for overcoming barriers and improving the translation of conventional research methods into community-based primary care settings is practice-based research networks (PBRNs) [2]. PBRNs conduct primary

This work was supported by grant award # 5R21HS013573-02 from the Agency for Healthcare Research and Quality and grant #049051 from the Robert Wood Johnson Foundation.

*Corresponding author. E-mail address: landerko@uwm.edu (L. Anderko).

0029-6465/05/$ – see front matter
doi:10.1016/j.cnur.2005.08.009

care research across primary health care delivery sites, which may be situated within at-risk communities, with a goal of delivering optimal, evidence-based health care within and across these communities. The Agency for Health care Research and Quality (AHRQ) was among the early federal supporters of PBRN research [3,4]. AHRQ defines a PBRN as: a group of ambulatory practices devoted principally to the primary care of patients, affiliated with each other (and often with an academic or professional organization) to investigate questions related to community-based practice [5].

AHRQ ascribes the following characteristics to PBRN research:

- Grounded in clinical and social sciences
- Emphasizes the complexities of conducting research in real-world settings and using secondary data
- Focuses on disseminating key research findings back into real-world practice and policy, and encouraging their implementation
- Addresses services that often are ignored in other medical or health services research, including mental health, dental, social, and enabling (ie, outreach services)
- May emphasize chronic care, acute care, or preventive care
- Includes studies of lifestyles and risk factors, and ways to change health behaviors [6]

In September 2000, AHRQ awarded grants to 19 PBRNs across the United States to help them enhance research in primary care settings. This initial group of federally funded primary care PBRNs provided access to over 5000 primary care providers and almost seven million patients in 49 states. As an expansion of this initiative, in 2002, AHRQ, through its Center for Primary Care Research, awarded developmental grants to increase the number of federally funded primary care PBRNs. AHRQ's overall goal with respect to PBRNs is to improve the capacity of PBRNs to expand the primary care knowledge base and to establish mechanisms that will assure that new knowledge is incorporated into actual practice and its impact assessed [6].

This article highlights the importance of PBRNs in primary health care research and underscores the need for community-based primary health research for addressing health disparities experienced by large populations in the United States. The unique community-based care delivered by nurses, in particular care delivered in community nursing centers (CNCs), provides a distinctive opportunity to combine the strengths inherent in CBPR methods and found within a PBRN to develop and test evidence-based practice that benefits health outcomes and decreases health disparities [7].

COMMUNITY NURSING CENTERS AS PRIMARY HEALTH CARE RESEARCH SITES

Nursing centers traditionally have served the health and illness needs of diverse populations of vulnerable urban and rural residents who are at risk for limited health care access and poor health outcomes [7]. CNCs provide a nontraditional model of primary health care delivery that has been developed over a 30-year period. CNCs frequently embrace the World Health Organization (WHO) definition of primary health care, which includes an emphasis on primary prevention, health promotion, and community empowerment [8]. These alternative models of primary health care delivery integrate traditional primary care, community health, public health, and social services, and include health promotion, disease prevention, health teaching, counseling services, intensive case management, and population-based programming in partnership with community organizations. Unlike traditional medical care venues that provide primary health care, and consistent with CBPR principles, CNCs emphasize community participation in program development, implementation, and evaluation [9].

CNCs typically are located in convenient locations where people live, work, learn, and play, making services readily available to community residents. CNC services are targeted to individuals and groups whose needs are not being met in the traditional delivery system. In many instances, the services provided by these CNCs are the only ones readily accessible to area residents. Collectively, these CNCs provide significant levels of primary health care to clients representative of every major racial group. Many CNC sites provide primary care management of illness for very low-income, underserved clients [9].

There is a paucity of research that provides evidence-based data related to the impact on the health of at-risk populations receiving care in CNCs that make use of unique, nursing models of health care delivery [10–14]. Health care providers, policy makers, and the communities served can benefit from the systematic study of:

- The structure and processes of primary health care provided by nurses to vulnerable populations in a community-based environment
- The impact on health care outcomes of the various models of care (traditional primary care, community-based nursing, public health) established in CNCs

Finally, evidence-based research studies are necessary to document primary health care practice and nurse-sensitive outcomes in CNCs to provide data that will define more clearly causal associations between nurse-delivered primary health care and the reduction of health disparities currently experienced by at-risk populations served by CNCs.

ESTABLISHING A NURSING PRACTICE-BASED RESEARCH NETWORK

PBRNs use the experience and insight of practicing clinicians to identify and frame research questions whose answers can improve the health outcomes of many populations, including the most vulnerable. They also provide a mechanism to produce research findings that are immediately relevant to clinicians and more easily assimilated into every day practice. The Committee on the Future of Primary Care, convened by the Institute of Medicine [15], has underscored the importance of PBRNs and described such networks as a promise for better science in primary care. Although multi-site research is not a new phenomenon, the idea of research networks in primary care takes multi-site research to a new level, particularly when focusing on primary health care delivery provided by nurses. In short, PBRNS for advanced practice nurses (APNs) and community nursing centers are a new phenomenon.

Tailored, community-based approaches that include multiple-level interventions have influenced health behaviors positively in the high-risk, ethnically diverse, low-income clients of CNCs. To reduce health disparities, it is imperative to conduct research in partnership with these communities to ensure that the interventions developed are culturally relevant, meaningful, and effective in changing lifestyles and health outcomes. This model of community participatory research can create clinical laboratories where the theories and practices of health and health care can be studied and evaluated in real-world settings for efficacy and effectiveness.

There is a critical need to include these populations and the primary health providers who serve them in clinical and health services research studies, if one is to gain insights into ways to improve their health status. CNCs also disproportionately serve minority populations and those at great risk for poor health outcomes, populations poorly represented in many research studies. Unfortunately, the unique potential for CNCs to serve as clinical laboratories for CBPR and health services research is mitigated, in part, by the fact that these nursing centers are typically quite small. To test interventions with a large enough sample size to allow statistical analysis and draw generalizations, multi-site studies are essential. Establishing a network of nursing centers can strengthen local research efforts by facilitating and supporting a synergistic team to carry out larger research studies and expanded programs of research. Nurse researchers can work collaboratively with community representatives to:

- Identify questions of significance to the populations served
- Plan and execute studies that include adequate numbers of participants from typically underrepresented populations
- Generate evidence that can be credibly translated back into best practices in CNC settings

THE MIDWEST NURSING CENTERS CONSORTIUM RESEARCH NETWORK

The Midwest Nursing Centers Consortium Research Network (MNCCRN) was funded by a grant from AHRQ in 2002 to begin developing a collaborative program of participatory community-focused research with vulnerable populations across multiple CNC sites. This research network began with 20 CNCs that had been in operation from 3 to 17 years and represented thirteen Midwestern universities (Lundeen, unpublished data, 2002). Several members were recruited into the network over the past 2 years. Unfortunately the fiscal instability of many of CNCs saw some members leave. As of spring 2005, the MNCCRN had 19 academic community nursing centers based in 15 universities in the Midwest.

The original purposes of the MNCCRN were to:

- Establish a practice-based research network for advanced nurse primary care providers who practice in nontraditional CNC settings
- Establish a Web-based system for data collection and transfer that will comply with evolving data privacy mandates
- To develop a collaborative program of participatory community-focused research with vulnerable populations that will inform primary care practice, health professional education, and health care policy (Lundeen, unpublished data, 2002).

Additionally, aims of the MNCCRN include linking with other nursing PBRNs and growing to a national network over time and generating new knowledge about CNC users, advanced nursing practice in community-based settings, and health outcomes among vulnerable and minority populations served by CNCs (Lundeen, unpublished data, 2002).

Finally, the overall strategy of the original grant was to support the expansion of several research programs undertaken by members. These research themes focus on:

- Interdisciplinary models of primary care service delivery that are accessible and culturally acceptable to vulnerable populations
- Practice models using clinical taxonomies incorporating nursing and medicine
- Implementation of an automated clinical documentation system that supports relational datasets for research
- Health outcomes measurement in a diverse client population
- Improvements in primary care through an environment of evidence-based practice and health policy advocacy (Lundeen, unpublished data, 2002).

METHODS: CREATING A RESEARCH INFRASTRUCTURE FOR THE MIDWEST NURSING CENTERS CONSORTIUM RESEARCH NETWORK

The process of creating a research infrastructure for the MNCCRN was built upon work established by the Midwest Nursing Centers Consortium (MNCC), a consortium of nursing centers located in the Midwest and established in 2001 with the purpose of collaborating on advocacy and research efforts. The organizational model developed for the MNCCRN is one that builds on long-standing relationships with community groups, other health care providers, and organizational linkages that will facilitate trust, increase communication, maximize the use of limited resources, and enhance the dissemination of new knowledge generated to multiple constituencies, including consumers, health professionals, and policy makers (Lundeen, unpublished data, 2002).

Each MNCCRN member agency has built into its infrastructure mechanisms for community input into the delivery of services and the implementation of research, with community advisory boards acting as the official mechanism for assuring community accountability of the centers. These boards include users of CNC services. Meetings are held throughout the year at each of the member sites. In addition to regularly scheduled meetings, consumer input is solicited through client satisfaction surveys that are conducted periodically at each center. The recent selection of a common tool to measure client satisfaction will allow the MNCCRN to conduct network-wide quality studies in the near future.

A MIDWEST NURSING CENTERS CONSORTIUM RESEARCH NETWORK RESEARCH STUDY EXEMPLAR: PRESCRIPTION FOR HEALTH, WELLNESS FOR A LIFETIME

The Robert Wood Johnson Foundation's Prescription for Health initiative provided funding for the MNCCRN's first research study. This study, Wellness for a Lifetime, took place in eight community nursing centers at seven universities in five states. The primary purposes of this research were to evaluate the outcomes of an accessible, culturally and educationally appropriate physical activity and nutritional intervention for high-risk, low-income, ethnically diverse clients of CNCs. A secondary purpose was to test the efficacy of conducting multi-site community-based intervention research in a network of CNCs. It proved to be a successful first test of the MNCCRN's ability to develop, implement, and evaluate research across the network (Table 1).

This project was designed to implement changes in behaviors of primary care providers and the clients they serve who are at high risk for chronic disease. The project focused on developing and implementing an intervention model that is appropriate for culturally diverse populations with limited access to primary care and at risk for very poor health outcomes. The study was designed to:

- Develop, implement and test strategies to improve the integration of health assessment and health promotion interventions intended to increase health-focused behaviors into standard primary care delivered to culturally diverse clients
- Implement and evaluate the impact of strategies designed to foster lifestyle changes for culturally diverse clients at risk because of sedentary lifestyle and unhealthy diet
- Determine potential and actual barriers to the care providers' integration of health assessments and health promotion referrals into standard primary care delivered to culturally diverse clients

The following goals were set forth for the project:

- Research/Wellness project implementation goal—to implement a research study and evaluate the MNCCRN research process through focus group discussions and client satisfaction surveys
- Provider behavior goal—to evaluate APN behaviors related to health assessment of physical activity, nutritional status, and associated risks, pre- and post-intervention, through use of chart audits and focus groups
- Client knowledge and behavior goals—to evaluate changes in client knowledge and behaviors related to physical activity and nutrition among participants in the 16-week Wellness for a Lifetime project, with an expectation

Table 1 Evaluation	Quantitative	Qualitative
Provider behavior goal	Pre- and postintervention chart audit of 25 client health records for the following elements during a well history and physical examination Client # Age Gender Race/ethnicity ICD9 codes Assessment of client's current nutrition status Assessment of client's current physical activity	Debriefing interviews were conducted among all project nurse practitioners regarding impact of project changes.
Implementation goal	Attendance at health education sessions	Posthealth education course evaluation tool, including: Classes Suggestions for improvement Barriers to implementation
Client knowledge and behavior goals	Pretest and post-test concerning: healthy eating and physical activity Weekly health diaries Weekly physical activity logs	Course evaluation for Satisfaction Changes in knowledge (pre- and posttest) Self analysis of changes in behavior related to improved nutrition and increased physical activity

that there would be improved knowledge or behavior of participants as a whole through pretest/post-test formats, food diaries, and satisfaction surveys (Anderko, unpublished data, 2004).

The APNs who staff the CNC study sites have an enduring passion and commitment to addressing issues facing vulnerable populations and reducing health disparities. Because this study was coordinated by CNC administrators and clinicians known to the target population, the MNCCRN research team had extensive access to and the trust of many individuals representing populations typically underrepresented in research studies. Study participants represented under- or uninsured men and women from Hispanic, African American, Native American and white racial and ethnic groups from urban and rural settings. Data collected for the study were entered into and stored in PBRNet, a Web-based, Health Insurance Portability and Accountability Act of 1996 (HIPAA)-protected data warehouse established by AHRQ (Anderko, unpublished data, 2004).

MAJOR FINDINGS

Self-reported behavior changes included increased movement or physical activity, and intake of a more balanced diet that included less junk food and more fruits and vegetables. In addition, APN assessment of physical activity and nutritional promotion increased. The following items highlight the major findings:

- Twenty-one APNs participated. Chart audits before and after the study found that APN assessment of physical activity levels (32.9% versus 47.5%) and nutritional status (30.5% versus 56.8%) improved significantly ($P < .01$).
- Clients were predominantly women (84%), with an age range between 25 and 83 years (mean could not be determined because of institutional review board [IRB] restrictions). The ethnic distribution was diverse, with African American (44.4%), white (44.4%), Hispanic (9.9%), and Native American (1.1%) participants.
- Of the 121 clients who signed consents, 82 started the program. Of those, 20 clients withdrew during the study, for an overall retention rate of 50%.

Overall knowledge scores for physical activity and nutrition improved ($P < .05$). Subjects relayed that they learned about health behaviors including: using stairs, how to live healthy and take care of self, increasing fiber, reducing sodium, and avoiding saturated fat, how to eat right, and the importance of activity and use of pedometers and diaries. Specifically, one subject stated there was an improvement in health behavior goal setting.

From the course evaluations, several comments reflected improved lifestyle behaviors. Subjects stated that they had begun to increase movement, activity, and exercise; were eating a more balanced diet with improved food choices, and others reported reducing junk food and increasing fruit and vegetable intake. Subject satisfaction surveys were submitted by 75.8% of course completers. The responses demonstrated very high satisfaction, with 63.8% of the respondents rating the course Excellent, 31.9% Very Good, and 4.3% Good. There were numerous comments about how good the course was, the quality of the instructors, and that the sessions and course should be longer. Other comments included; "How wonderful of you to be concerned about my health," and "The program saved my life" (Anderko, unpublished data, 2004).

Collaboration and cooperation between the CNCs were essential to getting the project completed, but these were challenging because of the geographic distances between the sites. Routinely meeting by means of video teleconferencing improved communication and collaboration efforts. Funding to support travel to these sites, however, would have been quite helpful and would have made the study stronger.

Another important consideration is that all CNCs are located within and have established partnerships with existing community agencies. Collaboration and cooperation between the CNCs and these agencies when conducting programs and research projects were vital to the success of this project. This study required that all CNCs located in various community agencies have this support. The good news is that these long-standing collaborative relationships between the eight CNCs and their community agency/sites supported research efforts.

RESEARCH NETWORK INFRASTRUCTURES: LESSONS LEARNED

There are significant challenges that must be addressed to sustain a synergistic, collaborative network for research. There must be a commitment to collaborative work across the network to articulate and implement programs of research. Ideally, priorities for research should be established and a clear assessment undertaken of the capabilities of each site and the network as a whole.

There must be constant vigilance maintained to identify research network funding opportunities. AHRQ-designated PBRNs are sometimes eligible for unique funding streams of given priority in other more general calls. Although there may be a centralized point for screening of funding opportunities appropriate for the network, this ongoing responsibility must be shared by representatives across the network to maximize the identification of potential sources of research support. Funding opportunities must be judged for their fit with the vision, mission, and purposes of the research network and the priority research agenda already established. Each call for proposals must be screened for feasibility in terms of individual site interests, abilities, costs, and client populations. The MNCCRN continues to strategize plans for responding to calls for proposals in a fashion that is expedient and receptive to research needs of the communities served by the various CNCs.

Ownership of data and dissemination plans need to be outlined during the initial phase of each study. Issues related to authorship determinations and plans for presentation at professional meetings need to be discussed and agreed upon as part of the collaborative effort. Shared authorship is encouraged to generate scholarly products that reflect the contributions of multiple members of the team while still maintaining rigorous standards for dissemination. The MNCCRN has agreed upon a standard for authorship determinations that clearly outlines responsibilities for each author.

Additional considerations include that the research network infrastructure must be developed and sustained through succeeding research grants. A large challenge for multi-site studies in nursing practice-based research networks is ensuring the consistency of the intervention across the sites and the reliability and validity of the data collected at each site. In the Wellness for a Lifetime project, consistency in the provision of the multi-dimensional intervention across sites so as to improve the reliability of the study findings was maximized through the use of video teleconferences. During video teleconferences, research team members were trained on the process, tools, and mechanisms for data collection. Questions and concerns were discussed by representatives of all sites so as to standardize the appropriate aspects of the intervention across research settings.

Although APNs are key managers and care providers at CNCs, it cannot be assumed that they can add the role of principal investigator or coinvestigator to their already substantial responsibilities. Nor should APNs be expected to be the sole recruiters of subjects, provide the research interventions, and collect the research data. To ensure consistency of intervention and reliability and validity of data, there must be a seasoned coinvestigator at each site who is ultimately responsible for each research study, in collaboration with CNC clinicians. Research coordinators and additional clinical staff to provide the intervention strictly according to protocol may need to be hired to conduct each study. Training and evaluation of the research team at each of the participating sites should be built into each proposal budget. Whenever possible, the principal investigator or the project director should plan to visit each participating site on a regular basis. Although travel funding sometimes is limited, these site visits can help to ensure the reliability and validity of the research study.

Communication among all research team members in the clinical sites has to begin as the protocol, additional documents and budget are being developed for submission to the funding agency. The principal investigator and the site coinvestigators need to agree upon clear, workable processes for subject recruitment and retention, delivery of the intervention, data collection, compilation, warehousing, and analysis and dissemination. Open and frequent communication mechanisms must be established. Conference calls, e-mail reflector lists, and video teleconferencing are all tools that can be used in lieu of face-to-face meetings.

A significant lesson learned by this PBRN during the first multi-site study was the variability in the IRB process across the seven university sites and the complexity in securing multiple institutional approvals. To facilitate the site coinvestigators' IRB submission processes, it is important that they are fully knowledgeable about the study protocol and budget. Ideally, IRB coordinators and chairs at each of the sites would agree to accept the principal investigator's IRB approval with minimal modifications.

SUMMARY

The evidence from the first MNCCRN study suggests that a shift in the level of wellness in a large percentage of the population of the nation may depend upon the ability to create new models of health care and promotion that merge the traditional model of primary care delivery with a public health approach to primary prevention and health promotion. Nurses can and must enter the field of CBPR using the power of community partnerships inherent in practice to integrate these principles into nursing research designs.

PBRNs provide important mechanisms for defining relevant research questions and acceptable research methods in partnership with community representatives, translating research into practice, improving health outcomes, and ultimately, changing health policy, based on evidence. There is great potential for teams of nurse clinicians and researchers to contribute to the discovery of new knowledge about innovative solutions to the complex problems of community practice and the health needs of diverse populations. In the future, MNCCRN plans to conduct a series of studies that can inform primary care practice with a special emphasis on interventions that can reduce the health disparities gap in many communities. Currently there are only two federally funded PBRNs nationwide that are anchored by APNs in primary care: MNCCRN and APRNet, a network of nurse practitioners in clinical settings throughout New England and coordinated by a team at Yale School of Nursing [16]. More nurse-anchored PBRNs must be established to provide leadership in reducing health disparities in this nation's neediest populations [17]. In the future, the MNCCRN will encourage and support the efforts of other regional PBRNs and seek to link with APRNet and emerging networks to create a national network of nurses conducting community-based participatory research in partnership with at-risk populations served by CNCs and other APNs. Such a network could have far reaching and significant impact on the health status of the populations nurses serve and the structure of health care delivery in the United States.

References

[1] Viswanathan M, Ammerman A, Eng E, et al. Community- based participatory research: assessing the evidence. Evidence report/Technology assessment No. 99 (Prepared by RTI-University of North Carolina Evidence-based Practice Center under contract No. 290–02–0016). AHRQ Publication 04–E022–2. Rockville (MD): Agency for Healthcare Research and Quality; 2004.

[2] Agency for Healthcare and Research Quality (AHRQ). Primary care: where research and practice meet. AHRQ. Available at http://www.ahrq.gov/about/cpcr/practice.pdf. Accessed January 10, 2005.

[3] North American Primary Care Research Group. Practice-based research networking for growing the evidence to substantiate primary care medicine. Ann Fam Med 2004;2: 180–1.

[4] Nutting PA, Green LA. Practice-based research networks: reuniting practice and research around the problems most of the people have most of the time. J Fam Pract 1994;38(4): 335–6.

[5] Primary care practice-based research networks. AHRQ Publication No. 01–P020. Agency for Healthcare Research and Quality. Available at www.ahrq.gov/research/pbrnfact.htm. Accessed November 14, 2004.

[6] Agency for Healthcare Research and Quality (AHRQ). Overview: Center for Primary Care Research. AHRQ. Available at www.ahrq.gov/abput/cpcr/cpcrover.htm. Accessed November 20, 2004.

[7] Pohl J, Vonderheid S, Barkauskas V, et al. The safety net: academic nurse-managed centers' role. Policy, Politics & Nursing Practice 2004;2(5):84–94.

[8] World Health Organization. Primary health care (WHO Alma Ata). Geneva (Switzerland): World Health Organization; 1978.

[9] Lundeen SP. An alternative paradigm for promoting health in communities: the Lundeen community nursing center model. Fam Community Health 1999;21(4):15–28.

[10] Anderko L, Robertson J, Uscian M. The effectiveness of a rural nursing center in improving health care access in a three-county area. J Rural Health 2000;16(2):177–84.

[11] Anderko L, Uscian M. Academic–community partnerships as a strategy for positive change in the sexual behavior of rural college-aged students. Nurs Clin North Am 2002;37(2): 341–9.

[12] Busen NH, Beech B. A collaborative model for community-based health care screening of homeless adolescents. J Prof Nurs 1997;13(5):316–24.

[13] Hildebrandt E, Baisch M, Lundeen S, et al. Eleven years of primary health care delivery in an academic nursing center. J Prof Nurs 2003;19(5):279–88.

[14] Anderko L, Uscian M. Quality outcome measures at an academic rural nurse-managed center: a core safety net provider. Policy, Politics & Nursing Practice 2001;2(4):288–94.

[15] Molla S, Donaldson KD, Yordy K, et al, editors. Primary care: America's health in a new era; Committee on the Future of Primary Care. Washington (DC): National Academy Press, Institute of Medicine; 1996.

[16] Grey M, Walker PH. Practice-based research networks for nursing. Nurs Outlook 1998;46(3):125–9.

[17] Flaskerud JH, Lesser J, Dixon E, et al. Health disparities among vulnerable populations: evolution of knowledge over five decades in nursing research publications. Nurs Res 2002;51(2):74–85.

Nurs Clin N Am 40 (2005) 759–770

NURSING CLINICS
OF NORTH AMERICA

ELSEVIER
SAUNDERS

Ethical Considerations for Nurse-Managed Health Centers

Susan M. Beidler, PhD, MBe, ARNP, BC

Quantum Foundation Center for Innovation in School and Community Well Being, Christine E. Lynn College of Nursing, Florida Atlantic University, 777 Glades Road, Boca Raton, FL 33431, USA

The current health care delivery system is complex and constantly changing. Increasing numbers of individuals have no health insurance coverage, as more employers drop benefits, and many low-wage workers remain ineligible for publicly funded health care programs. Subsequently, many people have difficulty accessing health care services [1]. Despite the lack of a clear mechanism for paying or providing the most basic level of health care for all, the national agenda for health care continues to emphasize increased access to quality health services [2,3]. The traditional health care delivery system has not made measurable gains toward meeting this goal. Unemployed and low-income populations are increasingly dependent upon community health centers and safety net providers for care. As one type of safety net provider, nurse-managed health centers (NMHCs) frequently care for populations with limited access to care [4]. NMHCs are prepared to address the needs of these populations and make progress toward meeting national health care goals [5,6].

NURSE-MANAGED HEALTH CARE: NOT A NEW SOLUTION

Throughout the post-Nightingale period, NMHCs have existed in various forms. From Lillian Wald's settlement houses to Margaret Sanger's birth control clinics and Mary Breckenridge's midwifery services, nurse activists have been at the forefront of addressing the unmet needs of individuals in the community [7]. These nurse activists sought to solve the twentieth-century problems caused by immigration, urbanization, and industrialization in the United States. The nurse practitioner movement in the mid-twentieth century expanded the role of the nurse to include primary care. Nurse practitioners (NPs), through their commitment to social justice, have become well-established primary care providers for vulnerable and marginalized patients and those at increased risk for poor health outcomes.

E-mail address: sbeidler@fau.edu

0029-6465/05/$ – see front matter
doi:10.1016/j.cnur.2005.08.008

ETHICAL NURSING PRACTICE

History illuminates nurses fulfilling their primary duty described in the Code of Ethics for Nurses: to practice "with compassion and respect for the inherent dignity, worth, and uniqueness of every individual, unrestricted by considerations of social or economic status, personal attributes, or the nature of health problems" [8]. Nurses and NPs may not always identify the Code of Ethics for Nursing as one of their guides for practice, but most will articulate their commitment to and advocacy for their patients [9]. The ethic of care that is integral to the practice of professional nursing is incorporated into the education and socialization of nursing. Public perception repeatedly has validated nursing as ethical through national surveys that consistently rank nursing as the most honest and ethical professions [10].

Nursing's professional commitment to ethical practice is challenged on a daily basis. Despite this nation's advanced democracy and technical ability, health disparities among millions of African Americans and other ethnic minorities continue to exist [11,12]. These disparities in health can be attributed directly to the inequities that exist in the health care delivery system. Many nurses struggle with these inequities, and some experience moral distress or burnout [13].

No group of patients suffers a wider health gap than blacks. In practically every type of illness and cause of preventable death but suicide, blacks suffer and die younger, faster, and at higher rates than whites [11,12]. As nurses attempt to uphold their commitment to treat all persons equally and unrestricted by considerations of social or economic status or personal attributes, moral conflict results. In so far as moral distress has been recognized as a consequence of nursing practice in ethically complex situations, little has been done to assist nurses with strategies to deal with this phenomenon.

Evidence supports that NMHCs meet the needs of multi-cultural and marginalized individuals who have difficulty accessing services [4]. In a 1998 American Association of Colleges of Nursing (AACN) survey, most nursing centers were situated in senior or neighborhood centers (25%), public housing projects (22%), community centers (16%), and shelters (15%). Culturally diverse patients made up 54% of the nursing centers' caseloads, comprised of patients who were non-English speaking (25%), homeless (19%), and mentally ill (8%). Persons over 85 years of age comprised 30% of the nursing centers' caseload. The National Nursing Centers Consortium (NNCC) reports that on average, 40% of the individual center's patients are uninsured (T. Hansen-Turton, personal communication, April 17, 2005).

ETHICAL CONSIDERATIONS

The increased number of individuals without insurance coverage, along with the evolution of Medicaid managed care, has created a practice environment rife with ethical issues. Many of the individuals cared for by nurses and NPs in NMHCs are vulnerable because of the increased relative risk or susceptibility to adverse health outcomes associated with being uninsured [14].

Vulnerable populations are those whose members are frequently marginalized from the center of society and as such are stripped of their voice, their power, and their rights to resources [15,16] . Poor health outcomes that frequently occur with vulnerable patients are increased morbidity, premature mortality, and diminished quality of life [17]. It is this combination of vulnerability, risk, and marginalization that contributes to the development of various ethical issues.

ETHICAL ISSUES IN NURSE-MANAGED HEALTH CENTERS
Many studies have been conducted for the purpose of identifying various ethical issues, conflicts, moral reasoning, and decision making used by professional nurses [18–25]. A few studies of NPs in ambulatory settings have been conducted [13,26,27]. Even fewer, however, have studied the nature and impact of ethical issues on primary care NPs caring for vulnerable patients [28,29]. Before discussing research related to NP practice, clarification of terminology frequently interchanged when discussing ethics is presented.

DILEMMAS, CONFLICTS, AND ISSUES
The language of ethics frequently uses the terms dilemma and conflict interchangeably. The dictionary definitions do not offer much clarification. A dilemma is defined as "an argument necessitating a choice between equally unfavorable or disagreeable alternatives; any situation in which one must choose between unpleasant alternatives; any serious problem" [30]. A conflict is defined as "a sharp disagreement or collision, as of interests or ideas, clash; emotional disturbance resulting from a clash of opposing impulses or from an inability to reconcile impulses" [30]. Davis and colleagues [31] define an ethical dilemma as existing when there are conflicting moral claims. Sullivan and colleagues [32] use this definition and then proceed to substitute the term conflict as they provide further description of ethical dilemmas. The terms conflict or dilemma represent a personal or individualized response to a situation that may or may not be duplicated (S.T. Fry, personal communication, February 7, 2001). Upon reflection of the definitions of conflict and dilemma, it can be seen that both involve choices that might be unfavorable, unpleasant, or emotionally disturbing. Arguably, what might be emotionally disturbing to one individual may not be to another. Moreover, not all ethically charged situations faced by primary care NPs reflect the possibility of a choice being made. Ethical issues tend to reflect particular types of nursing practice. The term issue is a more inclusive term and more appropriately used when evidence of a choice is not immediately evident. Published studies use all three terms. The terms selected for specific studies may or may not have significance; therefore their use needs to be considered when reading results.

Dilemmas
Viens' [12] study of moral dilemmas experienced by NPs in primary care settings found that most categories of dilemmas were situated around client issues related to themes of maleficence versus beneficence, rights versus

responsibilities, and justice. An example of a dilemma categorized as beneficence versus maleficence related to the NP attempting to make a decision about
referring a patient to a research protocol in which there was the possibility of
the patient receiving placebo versus medication. The NP was not comfortable
with the thought that by referring the patient to the research protocol, he might
receive the placebo instead of just getting customary care. Another NP in the
study described the dilemma of deciding between a patient's right to privacy
about his infectious disease status and the public's right to protection, which
was categorized as an example of patient rights versus professional responsibility. Dilemmas related to justice occurred when the NP wrestled with her need
to make an income for herself, generate an income for the clinic, and still provide quality care for patients who were uninsured.

After identifying dilemmas such as these, Viens [33] also examined the processes used to resolve the dilemmas. She found that NPs used a complex process of critical thinking that began with the clinical decision making process.
She also noted that values were identified in the various courses of action. Values, defined as personal ideals that motivated the individuals in making decisions and choosing the courses of actions surrounding the moral dilemma,
revolved around the NP's relationship with the patient. Values identified by
Viens were: responsibility, caring, respect for persons, respecting confidentiality, justice, rights/access to health care, trust, honesty, helping, sanctity of life,
religious beliefs, empathy, beneficence, and intuitive values. Caring, the value
mentioned by most of the NPs, was seen as the thing that nurses do and do
well, and was perceived as empowering nursing to evolve into a special relationship with clients to be therapeutic. The client was identified as an individual
or society, and relationship was defined as a purposeful, therapeutic interaction.

Viens' 1994 study categorized the dilemmas and values experienced by primary care NPs. The study emphasized that influencing factors were of para-
mount importance, because they changed the context of a situation from an
ordinary everyday clinical encounter to a moral dilemma. Several influencing
factors identified in this study were the practice setting, the operation of the
Medicaid system, and the recruitment of patients into research protocols that
included performing painful tests required for monitoring the patient during
a drug study. The study supported theory that identifies woman's morality
as contextual instead of objective [34,35]. Viens made a strong case for implementing ethics instruction in primary care NP educational programs and for
focusing discussions at regional NP meetings on how to avert or resolve moral
dilemmas.

Turner and colleagues [29] identified the types of ethical dilemmas encountered by rural primary care NPs and identified constraints and enhancers that
influenced their ethical decision making. Patients in rural settings frequently
shared the characteristics of being poor and vulnerable with urban-residing patients. The authors interviewed nine NPs, and analysis resulted in the identification of eight types of situations that resulted in ethical dilemmas. These
included: patient noncompliance, abortion, immunizations, teen pregnancy,

financial constraints interfering with care, confidentiality, regulations/rules/laws, and incompetence of other health professionals. Similar to Viens [13], Turner and colleagues identified conflicts involving the principles of beneficence, maleficence, and justice. In addition, they identified the principle of autonomy as involved in dilemmas associated with abortion, immunization, and teen pregnancy.

Conflicts

Butz and colleagues [26] explored ethical conflicts experienced by pediatric NPs in ambulatory settings. The conflicts were analyzed according to an a priori four-category classification system for content analysis. This system included:

- Practice context of the conflict
- Principles and values that have commonly understood meaning and their conflict with other ethical principles and norms
- How the conflict was experienced using Jameton's definitions of moral conflicts in nursing practice
- Resolution of the conflict

The first classification (context of the ethical conflict) for most responses was the parent/child/practitioner relationship (34%). This included such circumstances as practitioner or patient disagreement with parents' treatment decisions, protection of child's rights, and protection of genetic/HIV/drug use information. The conflicts that occurred with greatest frequency with regard to the second classification (norms or principles) were related to contraception/abortion/sexually transmitted disease treatment (15%). A conflict between the principles of beneficence and nonmaleficence was identified with the next greatest frequency (12%). The third classification (type of conflict experienced, such as dilemma, distress, or uncertainty) identified conflicts as occurring 31% of the time. A conflict existed when principles or values conflicted with other ethical principles or other ethical norms. Most ethical conflicts (22%) were not resolved, as identified in the fourth classification system. The authors of this study called for further research on the impact of unresolved conflicts on patient care and outcomes and supported the need for mechanisms by which ethical conflicts can be resolved.

In a clinical article about primary care NPs and nurse midwives (NMs) [36], Wurzbach discussed the moral conflicts posed by managed care. Although this was not an empirical study, it offered an interesting perspective on the virtue of justice as it applies to NPs and NMs. Wurzbach suggested that nurses and physicians need to function as double agents, that is, as providers who are simultaneously agents of the patient and the insurance carrier, hospital, or practice plan, and that this creates a series of ethical conflicts. She believed that NPs and NMs are the nurses most directly affected by health care reform in an ethical sense and identified that a resolution to this conflict would be to have justice with integrity. Justice with integrity is described as treating persons in like circumstances similarly, attempting to influence public policy with regard to distribution of benefits and burdens, making sure that patients understand their insurance benefits, and considering the fairness of policies. The author suggested that if doctors and nurses practice justice with integrity, they would protect all of society from distrust and cynicism directed at health care practitioners.

ETHICAL DECISION MAKING
The study by Turner and colleagues [29] contributed to nursing and ethical knowledge in that it addressed factors that constrain or enhance ethical decision making. Constraints were identified as rules and regulations, time, conflicts with physicians and other health care providers, past experiences, emotional closeness to the patient, limited or inadequate patient information, isolation of peers and facilities, and difficult decision making. Good rapport with clients, support from peers and mentors, access to a referral system, rules and regulations, prior experiences, intuition, emotional remoteness, client involvement, and holistic understanding of the client were identified as enhancers of ethical decision making. This study reinforced the importance that other authors have placed on clarifying one's personal values in the process of making ethical decisions [19,37].

In reviewing the extant literature on nurse practitioners and NMHCs, it was determined that the ethical issues experienced in NMHCs caring for vulnerable patients had not been the focus of any study. To address this knowledge gap, Beidler [9] conducted a naturalistic inquiry aiming to obtain more significant and specific knowledge about the ethical issues experienced by NPs caring for vulnerable populations in NMHCs and how they were handled by the NP.

ETHICAL ISSUES
This purposeful participant sample of NPs was selected from not-for-profit NMHCs affiliated with a consortium of nursing centers in the mid-Atlantic region of the United States. An effort was made to obtain the widest variety of NPs, ethical issues, and practice settings available. In other words, NPs from various programs (family, pediatric, and adult), encountering various types of ethical issues, and from various types of centers (free-standing, university-affiliated, and hospital-affiliated) and practice settings (rural and urban) were selected. Additional effort was made to select participants who had practiced as NPs for a minimum of 2 years, excluding their student clinical experience. This period of time was identified in an effort to select NPs who were competent in their practice. Competence, as described by Benner [38], develops when a nurse has been on the same or similar job for 2 to 3 years, and when she can base a plan of care on conscious, abstract, and analytic contemplation of a problem.

Observations of practice settings, intensive interviews of NPs, and document collection were the major methods of data collection. The NPs were asked to complete a brief demographic survey that provided information about their education, years of experience, practice setting, and patient population. Open-ended questions were used to elicit the emic perspective of the ethical issues experienced by primary care NPs. Field notes were completed; these recorded details of observations, encounters, practice environments, and other events. Documents were collected, organized, and analyzed. Documents included mission statements, practice brochures, policies, procedures, guidelines, memos, statutes, and rules and regulations that impacted the NP's practice or practice setting. Through the process of comparative analysis, data from subsequent cases were compared with the previous cases, and ideas, events, or acts that shared common characteristics were labeled with the same codes and categories.

Eleven primary care NPs participated in the study. Only one NP was educated as an adult NP, with the remainder educated as family NPs. They averaged 8.8 years of experience, ranging from 1 year to 31 years. They worked at their current practice sites for an average of 5.4 of years. Most (n = 9) of the programs from which the NPs graduated were masters level. Two completed postmasters NP programs. All but one NP responded that she had taken an ethics course or had ethics content integrated into the curriculum at some point in her overall nursing education. Seven NPs stated that they did not have ethics consultation available to them at their NMHCs.

Ten primary care NMHCs were the settings for the study. The centers were categorized by size, setting, affiliation, and patients. Centers with one to two employees were categorized as small, three to four employees as medium, and five or more as large. The NP participants were asked to categorize their settings as urban, suburban, or rural. Centers were categorized as being affiliated with a multi-service social agency (MSSA), hospital, university, or a joint venture of any of these.

Most NMHCs were small in size (n = 4), with an equal number of medium (n = 3) and large centers (n = 3). They were typically located in urban settings (n = 6). Two of the nursing centers were located in rural settings and two others in suburban settings. Most nursing centers (n = 3) were affiliated with an MSSA, a large social service corporation of which the nursing center is one of several services. Two centers were affiliated with hospitals and two with universities. The other three nursing centers had joint agreements, one between a university and another community health center, a second one between a university and a hospital, and the third between a free-standing center and university. Thus, half (n = 5) of all nursing centers were in some way affiliated with a university.

All of the NMHCs were established to provide comprehensive primary health care services. Social services either were provided on site or upon referral to an affiliated agency. Three of the centers provided comprehensive behavioral health services in addition to primary health care services. Community education, support groups, and outreach services were provided by most of the nursing centers. Two of the centers operated vans for transporting patients to appointments and conducting various outreach services.

Various patients were cared for in these NMHCs. All of the centers cared for patients of all genders and ages. Most patients in four of the centers were African American. The patients in two centers were primarily Hispanic or Latino. Two other centers' patients were primarily white. The patients in the two final centers were primarily African American and Hispanic. One of these centers provided services solely for homeless people.

A theme began to emerge early in the analysis of data. While analyzing the descriptions of the various ethical issues NPs experienced and handled, it became apparent that the issues were occurring at different levels within the sociopolitical context of delivering health care, resulting in issues seeming to cluster at different levels. Thus, the Beidler Levels of Ethical Issues Framework was derived inductively while contemplating the range and level of issues that NPs identified and what they did about them. Further conceptualization and development of the framework were based on the researcher's perspective of the sociopolitical context within which these ethical issues occurred.

BEIDLER LEVELS OF ETHICAL ISSUES FRAMEWORK
Level one issues
Several ethical issues were indicative of situations that occurred directly between the patient and the NP. These issues involved the patient–NP relationship, the NPs personal philosophy of care or nursing, the NP's sense of self (personal knowing), the moral view of the patient, and the values of the patient or NP. As the participants described why they identified certain issues as ethical or why they were disturbing to them, it was evident that they resulted directly from the interaction between the patient and NP and not from any other sociopolitical structure. This relationship was identified as the patient–NP covenant. Ethical issues that related to the patient–NP relationship were categorized as level one.

The significance of level one issues was that handling these issues was within the sphere of influence of the NPs. In other words, resolution of the conflict or issue is possible through direct communication or interaction with the patient.

Level two issues
The next level of ethical issues seemed to result from a conflict between the NPs views, values, beliefs, or ethics and those of the NMHC administrators or other staff within the center. These issues were categorized as intra-agency issues. Level two ethical issues also might occur as a result of conflict between the NP or NMHC and an affiliated or sponsoring agency. These issues were coded as interagency issues. Additional conflicts might occur between the NP and her profession, such as with a lack of agreement between the NP and the Nurse Practice Act, Code of Ethics, or Nightingale Pledge. These were coded as intradisciplinary.

Ethical issues that occurred at level two went beyond the NPs' immediate sphere of influence or power to control. For example, if the issue occurred because of a conflict between the NP and the affiliated agency, it most likely required more than simply communication between the two parties. It might require writing letters to agency representatives or it might require bringing other NPs, staff members, or patients into dialog with the agency to make a change and resolve the issue. If the issue is not immediately resolvable, it might require additional staff support or education to address the areas where the conflict or issue existed.

Level three issues

Ethical issues that occurred at this level involved a conflict between the NP and another profession. For example, level three issues occurred when the NP was in conflict with the collaborating physician or a specialist to whom a patient had been referred. These types of conflicts seem to occur because of mismatched professional practice acts or codes of ethics. Another example is a situation that occurred when a physician refused to treat a patient because of the patient's inability to pay, which was in direct conflict with the NP's code of ethics. Ethical issues such as this were coded as interdisciplinary. Other ethical issues that were categorized as level three were those that resulted from a conflict between agencies, not directly affiliated with the NP or her agency, but with which the NP needed to interact on behalf of a patient. These were coded as extra-agency issues. The final types of issues at this level are those that occurred between two distinct professions other than nursing and impacted patient care. These were coded extradisciplinary. An example of this type of issue would be conflict between a physician and pharmacist that might interfere with a patient receiving a needed medication.

Level three issues were even more difficult to handle, because they were totally outside the NPs professional sphere of influence. Resolution of issues at this level required that the individual NP had the support of the profession or some other organizational structure to enhance the power base.

Level four

Ethical issues that involved conflicts with statutes or rules and regulations were the most difficult to resolve. An example of an issue at this level was patients' ineligibility for government-sponsored insurance programs (Medicare or Medicaid) unless the patient was, generally speaking, old, poor, or disabled. The only way to resolve ethical issues at this level was to influence the legislative or regulatory process.

The Beidler Levels of Ethical Issues Framework provides a mechanism for understanding where ethical issues commonly occur while caring for vulnerable patients in NMHCs. It offers a structure for educating NP students and practicing NPs as to the amount of control they might have over influencing the outcome of the issue. With this added knowledge, NPs have a framework by which to recognize and handle frequently occurring ethical issues and hopefully decrease the development of moral distress.

ETHICAL CONSIDERATIONS RELATED TO MANAGED CARE

NMHC centers have been successful in their negotiations with managed care organizations. Managed care plans are commonplace in the for-profit insurance world. More recently, Medicaid and Medicare programs have been integrated into this method of payment. Ulrich and colleagues [39] explored predictors of

NP autonomy in a managed-care environment. In their survey of 254 NPs certified and licensed in Maryland, they found that even though NPs were concerned about their autonomy, their autonomy scores remained high. Additionally, their study was unable to support the notion that managed care is a more unethical system than fee-for-service.

Ulrich and colleagues [40] also reported the ethical conflicts experienced by NPs in a managed care environment. In this report, they identified that most NPs responded that they were moderately to extremely concerned with managed care and that a large number of NPs (61%) identified that it was sometimes necessary to bend managed care guidelines to act in the patient's best interest.

SUMMARY

NMHCs have been in existence in one form or another for more than 100 years. The passion shared by visionary nurses who started the early centers is similar to that which continues to impassion nursing leaders today, that is, the desire to improve the human condition. Significant contributions to meeting quality health care needs of the nation have been made by NMHCs [41–43]. Numerous studies have shown the significant impact that nurse practitioners have had also [44–46]. Inherent in caring for most patients in NMHCs is the need to make moment-to-moment clinical decisions. It is frequently difficult to differentiate nursing clinical decision making from ethical decision making. That is because every nursing situation is an ethical situation. Nurses and NPs need to acknowledge the symbiosis of ethics and nursing.

It has been suggested that NPs should have their own code of ethics, since the role of the NP is unique [47]. The uniqueness of the NP role in the health professional circle is definitely apparent, particularly because the scope of practice goes beyond that of other professional nurses prepared at the baccalaureate level. However, an ethical code as a system of principles and rules reflects the rights and responsibilities of a profession and sets standards to regulate the conduct of practitioners of nursing. NPs grounded in the practice of nursing first and foremost and subsequently practicing in an expanded nursing role are guided appropriately by the American Nurses Association Code of Ethics for Nurses. Developing a separate code for NPs is incongruent with the purpose of professional codes.

Energy would be spent better educating NPs about ethical considerations when caring for patients in NMHCs. As patient advocates, students and practicing nurses and NPs alike must develop the skill to assist their patients during ethically charged situations, such as withdrawing of life support or deciding the direction of an unplanned pregnancy. Strategies for assisting NPs in addressing ethical issues must be developed also. Ethics committees from within the NMHCs, nearby acute care institutions, or community-based ethics consortia must be made available to nurses and NPs in NMHCs to have a mechanism to address their concerns. When the ethics committee structure does not exist, access to an ethics consultant would be beneficial to nurses and patients alike. In Beidler's [9] study on ethical issues caring for vulnerable patients, several of the NP participants expressed appreciation for being asked to participate. These NPs stated that the process of being interviewed for the study was almost like ethical therapy, suggesting therapeutic effects of qualitative research methods and the benefit of having someone with whom to discuss ethically or morally distressful practice situations.

It is difficult to predict the future of NMHCs in the current health care delivery system. These centers are clearly at the crossroads of needs and services, and they are accessible to those who need services the most. Nurses, NPs, and NMHCs have the potential to greatly influence the health care delivery system and this nation's health. Revising federal guidelines for expanding payment to NMHCs centers would be a notably ethical thing to do.

References
[1] Steinbrook R. Disparities in health care—from politics to policy. N Engl J Med 2004;350: 1486–8.
[2] United States Department of Health and Human Services. Developing objectives for healthy people 2010. Washington, DC: United States Department of Health and Human Services; 1997.
[3] Andrulis DP. Access to care is the centerpiece in the elimination of socioeconomic disparities in health. Ann Intern Med 1998;129:412–6.
[4] Pohl JM, Vonderheid SC, Barkauskas VH, et al. The safety net: academic nurse-managed centers' role. Policy, Politics & Nursing Practice 2004;5:84–94.
[5] Barger SE. Academic nursing centers: the road from the past, the bridge to the future. J Nurs Educ 2004;43:60–5.
[6] Benkert R, Pohl JM, Coleman-Burns P. Creating cross-racial primary care relationships in a nurse-managed center. J Cult Divers 2004;11:88–99.
[7] Glass LK. The historic origins of nursing centers. NLN Publ 1989;(21-2311):21–33.
[8] American Nurses Association. Code of ethics for nurses with interpretive statements. Washington, DC: American Nurses Publishing; 2001.
[9] Beidler SM. Ethical issues experienced by primary care nurse practitioners caring for vulnerable patients in nursing centers. Philadelphia, PA; 2002.
[10] Moore DW. Nurses top list in honesty and ethics poll. Available at: http://www.gallup.com/poll/content/login.aspx?ci=14236. Accessed April 2, 2005.
[11] Centers for Disease Control and Prevention. Health disparities experienced by black or African Americans—United States. MMWR Morb Mortal Wkly Rep 2005;54:1–3.
[12] Centers for Disease Control. Health disparities experienced by Hispanics, United States. MMWR Morb Mortal Wkly Rep 2004;36:935–7.
[13] Viens DC. Moral dilemmas experienced by nurse practitioners. Nurse Pract Forum 1994;5: 209–14.
[14] Flaskerud JH, Winslow BJ. Conceptualizing vulnerable populations, health-related research. Nurs Res 1998;47:69–78.
[15] Hall JE, Stevens PE, Meleis AI. Marginalization: a guiding concept of valuing diversity in nursing knowledge development. ANS Adv Nurs Sci 1994;16:23–41.
[16] Meleis AI. Culturally competent scholarship: substance and rigor. ANS Adv Nurs Sci 1996;19:1–16.
[17] Rogers AC. Vulnerability, health and health care. J Adv Nurs 1997;26:65–72.
[18] Allmark P. The ethical enterprise of nursing. J Adv Nurs 1992;17:16–20.
[19] Borawski DB. Resources used by nursing administrators in ethical decision making. Journal of Nursing Administrators 1994;24:17–22.
[20] Bunting SM, Webb AA. An ethical model for decision making. Nurse Pract 1988;13: 30–4.

[21] Carpenter M. The process of ethical decision making in psychiatric nursing practice. Issues Ment Health Nurs 1991;12:179–91.

[22] Grundstein-Amado R. Ethical decision-making processes used by health care providers. J Adv Nurs 1993;18:1701–9.

[23] Kelly B. Preserving moral integrity: a follow-up study of new graduate nurses. J Adv Nurs 1998;28:1134–45.

[24] Millette BE. Client advocacy and the moral orientation of nurses. West J Nurs Res 1993;15: 605–74.

[25] Wilkinson JM. Moral distress in nursing practice: experience and effect. Nurs Forum 1988;23:16–29.

[26] Butz AM, Redman BK, Fry ST. Ethical conflicts experiences by pediatric primary care nurse practitioners in ambulatory settings. J Pediatr Health Care 1998;12:183–90.

[27] Murphy C. Levels of moral reasoning in a selected group of nursing practitioners. New York: Teachers College, Columbia University; 1977.

[28] Maher PL, White PA. Ethical decision making in advanced nursing with community-dwelling elders. Clin Excell Nurse Pract 1997;1:423–7.

[29] Turner LN, Marquis K, Burman ME. Rural nurse practitioners: perceptions of ethical dilemmas. J Am Acad Nurse Pract 1996;8:269–74.

[30] Webster's new world college dictionary. New York: Macmillan; 1997.

[31] Davis AJ, Aroskar MA, Liaschenko J, et al, editors. Ethical dilemmas and nursing practice. 4th edition. Stamford (CT): Appleton & Lange; 1997.

[32] Sullivan E, Fields B, Kelly J, et al. Nursing centers: the new arena for advanced practice nursing. In: Mezey MD, McGivern DO, editors. Nurses, nurse practitioners. 2nd edition. New York: Springer; 1993. p. 251–64.

[33] Viens DC. The moral reasoning of nurse practitioners. J Am Acad Nurse Pract 1995;7:277–85.

[34] Gilligan C. In a different voice. Cambridge (MA): Harvard University Press; 1982.

[35] Gilligan C. In a different voice: psychological theory and women's development. Cambridge (MA): Harvard University Press; 1993.

[36] Wurzbach ME. Managed care: moral conflicts for primary health care nurses. Nurs Outlook 1998;46:62–6.

[37] Raines DA. Values influencing neonatal nurses' perceptions and choices. West J Nurs Res 1994;16:675–91.

[38] Benner P. From novice to expert: excellence and power in clinical nursing practice. Boston, MA: Addison Wesley Publishing Company; 1984.

[39] Ulrich CM, Soeken KL, Miller N. Predictors of nurse practitioners' autonomy: effects of organizational, ethical, and market characteristics. J Am Acad Nurse Pract 2003;15:319–25.

[40] Ulrich CM, Soeken KL, Miller N. Ethical conflict associated with managed care: views of nurse practitioners. Nurs Res 2003;52:168–75.

[41] Edwards JB, Kaplan A, Barnett JT, et al. Nurse-managed primary care in a rural community: Outcomes of five years of practice. Nursing and Health Care Perspectives 1998;19:20–5.

[42] Lenehan GP, McInnis BN, O'Donnell D, et al. A nurses' clinic for the homeless. Am J Nurs 1985;85:1237–40.

[43] Riesch SK. A primary care initiative: nurse-managed centers. In: Mezey MD, McGivern DO, editors. Nurses, nurse practitioners. Boston: Little-Brown; 1985. p. 242–8.

[44] Brown SA, Grimes DE. A meta-analysis of nurse practitioners and nurse midwives in primary care. Nurs Res 1995;44:332–9.

[45] Mundinger MO, Kane RL, Lenz ER, et al. Primary care outcomes in patients treated by nurse practitioners or physicians: a randomized trial. JAMA 2000;283:59–68.

[46] US Congress Office of Technology Assessment. Nurse practitioners, physician assistants, and certified nurse midwives: a policy analysis (health technology case study). Washington (DC): US Government Printing Office; 1986.

[47] Peterson M, Potter RL. A proposal for a code of ethics for nurse practitioners. Journal of the American Academy of Nurse Practitioners 2004;16:116–24.

Nurs Clin N Am 40 (2005) 771–778

NURSING CLINICS
OF NORTH AMERICA

The Collaboration of Public Health Nursing and Primary Care Nursing in the Development of a Nurse Managed Health Center

Anne Ferrari, PhD, RN*, Barbara Rideout, MSN, APRN, BC

Drexel University College of Nursing and Health Professions, 1505 Race Street, Mail Stop 501, Philadelphia, PA 19102, USA

The early 1990s was a time of great expectation for substantial change in health care delivery. A senator from Pennsylvania had been elected on a platform of health care reform, and it was a strong theme in the election of President Bill Clinton. Nurse practitioner programs were developed in many colleges and universities to meet the demands of the proposed new health care delivery system. Nurse-managed health centers (NMHCs) were springing up across the country, providing services from health promotion, to screening, to primary care. It seemed like a great way to get desperately needed services to populations with limited access. The dilemma became how to financially provide these services, because nurses were not readily reimbursable.

Until 1996, nursing education at Drexel University, then known as MCP Hahnemann University, existed as a department within the School of Health Professions. In 1996, however, recognizing the importance of nursing in the ever changing health care delivery system, the Department of Nursing gained academic recognition as a school, taking its place in the university next to the Schools of Health Professions, Medicine, and Public Health. In July 2000, the College of Nursing and Health Professions was formed by the merger of the School of Nursing and the School of Health Professions. This created an opportunity for expanded community outreach initiatives under the leadership of Dr. Patricia Gerrity, associate dean for community programs. Specifically, a collaborative relationship with the Philadelphia Housing Authority (PHA) to deliver on-site health care to four PHA housing facilities was established. One neighborhood, known as the 11th Street Corridor, suffered with a heavier burden of morbidity and mortality than other sections of Philadelphia and became the focused target. In an eight-block area, there were four public housing developments with a dense population of medically underserved clients. This

*Corresponding author. *E-mail address*: af33@drexel.edu (A. Ferrari).

0029-6465/05/$ – see front matter © 2005 Elsevier Inc. All rights reserved.
doi:10.1016/j.cnur.2005.08.006   nursing.theclinics.com

community served as the basis of focus groups, which were conducted at various sites in the 11th Street Corridor during the late 1990s. This initiative was unique, because on-site practices were developed by public health nurses (PHNs), while other nurse-managed centers were being established throughout the country by nurse practitioners and academicians.

This article discusses the collaboration of public health nursing and primary care nursing in the development of the 11th Street Family Health Center, a nurse-managed family health center located in Philadelphia. The first section defines the authors' view of the roles of public health nursing, primary care nursing, and preventive health services in underserved communities. The second section describes the developmental process of the initial public health nursing practice and primary care practice established with the community. The third portion addresses the collaboration between the PHNs and nurse practitioners as a cornerstone in the development of the 11th Street Family Health Center. The article concludes with a discussion of the some of the lessons learned in the development of one nurse-managed health center that was grounded in the collaboration of public health nursing practice and nurse practitioner practice.

THE ROLE OF PUBLIC HEALTH NURSING

PHNs work in schools, homes, clinics, jails, shelters, out of mobile vans, and on dog sleds. They are expert at working with communities, the individuals and families that compose those communities, and the systems that impact the health of those communities. They use a core set of interventions to accomplish their goals. Public health interventions are population-based by focusing on entire populations possessing similar health concerns or characteristics. Population-based care always begins by identifying everyone who is at-risk (ie, all children who can be immunized against vaccine-preventable disease) [1].

Public health interventions are guided by an assessment of the population health status through a community health assessment process. Public health nurses identify risk factors, health problems, protective factors, and assets of the population. The practice focuses on the entire range of factors that determine health, not just personal health risks or disease, but also income, housing, nutrition, employment, working conditions, social supports, education, safety and violence issues, cultural customs and values, and the community's capacity to support family and economic growth [2].

Public health nursing interventions consider all levels of prevention, but with a preference for primary prevention. This approach is very different from the medical model, in which people seek treatment when they are ill or injured. These interventions consider all levels of practice and are individual/family focused, community-focused, and systems-focused [1,2].

At the individual/family level, PHNs counsel women and men regarding their risk for sexually transmitted disease (STD) and prevention measures. Community-focused interventions include screening and surveillance. For example, PHNs operate a STD testing site targeting populations at risk for STDs. In addition to screening for diseases, they provide health teaching and counseling during the assessment. At a systems level, PHNs negotiate with local family planning services to routinely screen all family planning clients for STDs and to provide treatment for those who have positive results from the PHN community screenings.

THE ROLE OF PRIMARY CARE PROVIDER

Primary care ideally is the point of access to health care. The role of the primary care provider (PCP) is to manage most of the patient's overall health care. It includes providing preventive services, assessment and diagnosis of health problems, coordination of visits to other health care providers as needed, and handling of emergencies. Primary care considers biologic, psychological, and social factors in the health of individuals, families, and communities. Primary care provides continuity of care over time. PCPs need to assume a sense of responsibility for the health of the community in which they provide care. Their role encompasses surveillance of health problems in the community and provision of health services to address these problems [3].

THE ROLE OF PREVENTIVE HEALTH SERVICES

A significant role of the PCP is to prevent disease and promote healthy lifestyles. Prevention measures are divided into primary, secondary, and tertiary levels. Primary measures include activities to prevent the onset of a given disease. The goal of primary prevention is to spare the suffering, burden, and cost associated with the disease. Examples include immunizations, chemoprophylaxis, and health-protecting education and counseling. Secondary prevention measures include activities to identify and treat asymptomatic persons who have risk factors for a given disease or who have preclinical disease. Examples include cancer screening, blood pressure monitoring, cholesterol measurement, and blood sugar measurement. Tertiary prevention measures are part of the management of persons with an established disease to minimize disease-associated complications and the negative health effects of the conditions. Examples of tertiary prevention include medication and lifestyle modifications to normalize blood glucose and treatment of hyperlipidemia in patients who have coronary heart disease [2].

DEVELOPING PUBLIC HEALTH NURSING PRACTICE IN THE COMMUNITY

This section describes the development of the initial public health nursing practices established within the community. The depiction of public health nursing practices is captured best in Virginia Henderson's classic definition of nursing:

"The unique function of the nurse is to assist the individual, sick or well, in the performance of those activities contributing to his health or recovery (or to peaceful death) that he would perform unaided if he had the necessary strength, will or knowledge, and to do this in such a way as to help him gain independence as rapidly as possible.... (The nurse) is temporarily the consciousness of the unconscious, the love of life for the suicidal, the leg of the amputee, the eyes of the newly blind, a means of locomotion for the infant, knowledge and confidence for the young mother, the (voice) for those too weak or withdrawn to speak [4]."

The authors' view of public health nursing is that which society does collectively to assure the conditions in which people can be healthy. As PHNs, the goal is to synthesize the art and science of public health and nursing.

The original practice sites for the 11th Street Family Health Center varied from a small two bedroom row home, to a church basement, to a community room in a senior residence. Initially, the authors' approach to their constituencies was through the vehicle of blood pressure checks. Hypertension is a serious health problem in this community, and taking blood pressure is safe and non-invasive, but most importantly, provides a strategy to know the people. As suspected, the blood pressure screens became a place where people could talk about the weather and social events and share concerns about many other issues, such as, how to pay the rent, how to connect with the food bank, or how to deal with community children on drugs.

THE BACKGROUND, PEOPLE, AND VISION

One guiding principle was starting where the people are, and during initial focus-group sessions, certain themes emerged. The people are low-income and predominantly African American. At these early focus-groups it became evident, that regardless of focus-group settings, the themes were consistent across church groups, community action groups, and PHA housing resident groups. It also became evident that the level of care and compassion exhibited in these focus groups was truly exemplary. The themes included, and were not limited to:

We are proud of our neighborhood and need more help for our children so that they do not start taking drugs.
- Many of our old timers need help getting food.
- Too many people get diabetes and then end up losing a foot or leg.
- Many people get strokes when they are in their 30s and 40s, and we need to help them.
- How can we prevent our young teenagers from becoming pregnant?
- We do not need more students from big universities doing surveys
- We do not need more people just coming to our neighborhood to ask us all kinds of questions and then leave.

These themes formed the basis of the authors' initial public health nursing practice, which was established in four PHA housing facilities, senior citizen's housing facilities located in the same community, and two separate Section 8 locations. The Section 8 programs provide rental assistance for low and very low income households by providing direct payments of rent through public housing authorities to landlords [5].

Four nursing faculty members who were highly experienced and funded practitioners formed the first public health nurse practice team. The initial vision was twofold: to establish a presence and to build trust. A community member was hired as an outreach worker to assist the PHNs in opening doors and minds in the community. The following case history provides one example of the early PHN intervention.

THE CASE HISTORY OF ALEXANDER M

Alexander was a tall handsome African American man who was in his 80s. He had served in the Army during World War II and quite proudly wore his veterans WWII cap while out in the neighborhood. He had lived in North Philadelphia all his life and was well respected in the community. He was a proud man, quiet, and very kind to others. Early one morning in February, he arrived at one of the authors' public health nursing sites and asked if anyone would be able to help him understand his medications. He initially had been evaluated and diagnosed with hypertension at a Veterans Administration (VA) hospital. The authors were able to monitor and help him maintain his blood pressure within normal limits.

During the next 2 years, he became a weekly visitor at the practice site and would have blood pressure checks, and if new medications were ordered, he would be interested in learning all about the new medications. The authors also consulted with his PCP at the VA hospital to clarify issues that arose. It became apparent that the social aspects of visiting the practice site were a strong reason for his attendance. He took great pride in telling his story about WWII when he was stationed in France and was most comfortable with the nursing students who rotated through the center. The students learned valuable history about the experience of black men who served in Europe during WWII.

As a respected member of the community, Alexander was also an important lay community leader who would refer community members to the practice site. He also kept the PHNs current and informed about neighborhood issues and became an important informal member of the team.

IMPLEMENTING PRIMARY CARE SERVICES

In the fall of 1998, it was determined that the public health teams had established credibility and a good relationship with the community and it was time to take the initiative to the next level. While the authors negotiated the building of a permanent health center, a temporary primary care site was set up in two rooms in one of the neighborhood community centers. Nurse practitioners from the faculty initially provided primarily episodic care. Earlier, Pennsylvania had implemented its Welfare to Work program, which involved placing all Medicaid-eligible patients in Southeast Pennsylvania into one of four health management organizations (HMO's). To be paid for providing care to this population, providers had to be credentialed by each HMO. That process was lengthy and continues to be daunting. At every step, there was another hurdle and one HMO, refused to include nurse practitioners in its panel of providers, despite state regulations to the contrary.

To provide a financial stream to support the practice, grants were written, and contracts were established with the Family Planning Council and Vaccines for Children through the city health department. The primary focus of the care provided was well adult and children's physicals and immunizations, gynecologic care, family planning options, STD screening and treatment, and management of chronic health problems such as hypertension and diabetes. In addition the authors participated in programs sponsored by the Regional Nursing Centers Consortium for lead poisoning and asthma.

Outreach workers and the PHNs continued to identify and refer patients needing care. In addition, they provided much of the health education support, offering classes on nutrition, exercise, diabetes management, cardiac care, well baby care, and other classes. The lead education program was done one-on-one in homes with babies under 2 years of age. Each family was given a bucket of cleaning supplies to reduce the amount of lead dust in their homes. The infants initially were screened at 9 months to 1 year of age, and more education about the role of diet in preventing lead poisoning was provided at that time. Home visits also were made to children with asthma who had had several emergency room visits. An environmental assessment was done, and families were provided with supplies and suggestions to reduce asthma triggers.

Simultaneously, the PHNs were conducting multiple health promotion programs in the community. One program, the Vial of Life, was conducted in senior residences and consisted of seniors placing a list of all current medications and essential health information in a plastic zip lock bag that was kept in their refrigerator. The PHNs collaborated with Emergency Medical Services of Philadelphia, and the program provided life-saving information should a senior become confused or unconscious and need to be transported to the hospital. The surrounding hospitals were alerted about the Vial of Life program.

Another program, The Prevention of Alcohol and Substance Abuse program, was conducted in multiple senior locations in conjunction with the Philadelphia Corporation on Aging. The three goals of this health promotion program were:

- To raise awareness on the problems of alcohol/substance use and abuse in older adult residents of selected PHA sites and senior residences
- To increase understanding and knowledge regarding physiologic changes in aging and the risk for use, misuse, and abuse of alcohol, street drug prescriptions, and over-the-counter medications in the elderly
- To enhance and develop support systems in the community that focus of alcoholism/substance use and abuse in older adults

The 11th Street corridor serves as a clinical site for undergraduate nursing students enrolled in Community Health Nursing course and for graduate students in other health related programs. Faculty and students conduct health fairs, influenza vaccine immunization outreach, after school health clubs, friendly visitor programs to homebound seniors. In addition, they provide support for grandparents raising grandchildren in a kinship caregiver program, and developed of the Community Arts and Theater Troup, which focuses on sensitive topics for middle school-age children (teen pregnancy and sexually transmitted infections).

As the primary care services grew, these programs by the PHNs served as a referral base. People in the community who were found on screening or interview to have health problems were able to see a nurse practitioner for a complete health assessment and management.

THE COLLABORATION OF PUBLIC HEALTH AND PRIMARY CARE

PHNs and primary care nurse practitioners working together to improve health care in a community is a logical partnership. PHNs are the eyes and ears of primary care in the community. Case finding through screening, outreach, surveillance, and disease/health event investigation identifies individuals and families with or at risk for illness or health problems. PHNs are the reason many individuals appear for care. They provide credibility for the primary care practice. PCPs are seen as authority figures, and patients often tell them what they want to hear. PHNs are trusted by members of the community. In addition, they can provide follow-up care for the visit in the form of case management—a gentle nudge for the patient who is unsure or frightened about the diagnosis and its impact. They provide valuable insight into the home situation and the real reasons why patients may not comply with medications and recommendations (ie, the address is empty lot, or there is no heat or running water).

LESSONS LEARNED

With hindsight being 20/20, the collaboration between public health nursing and primary care provided the perfect marriage of the two disciplines. PHNs paved the road into the community, assessed the specific needs of the community, and established a level of trust that is unmatched. It is much like the experiences that occur during courtship and the engagement period in a relationship. Once the 11th Street Family Health Center was ready to provide primary care services, PHNs entered that portion of the relationship with eyes open and with all the nuances of the newly married very obvious. The result is a nurse-managed health center that has worked with the community which it serves, provided care that is urgently needed, and addressed the community's issues. From the perspective of the providers, insight was gained into the needs identified by the community. The authors had been told, "Just set it up and they will come." That has been true, but they were able to build a building that houses not just primary care and outreach services, but dental, physical therapy, and behavioral health services. In addition, the 11th Street Family Health Center offers a place for community groups to meet, a nutrition center, a designated food giveaway program, and classrooms for the community and university groups. The partnership with the people of the community is unsurpassed by others who have tried unsuccessfully to accomplish similar objectives. The authors believe that the collaboration of PHNs and the nurse practitioners is an excellent way to provide much needed services to this vulnerable population.

References

[1] St. Paul Minnesota Department of Health Public Health Nursing Section. Public health interventions—applications for public health nursing practice. St. Paul (MN): St. Paul Minnesota
Department of Public Health Nursing Section; 2001.

[2] Stanhope M, Lancaster J. Community and public health nursing. St. Louis (MO): Mosby, Incorporated; 2004.

[3] Dunphy LM. Primary care: the art and science of advanced practice nursing. Philadelphia: FA
Davis; 2001.

[4] Sitzman K, Eichelberger L. Understanding the work of nurse theorists: a creative beginning.
Boston: Jones and Bartlett; 2005.

[5] Wells Fargo Brokerage Products on-line glossary. Available at: http://www.wellsfargo.com/
wfcra/glossary.jhtml. Accessed February 21, 2005.

Nurs Clin N Am 40 (2005) 779–790

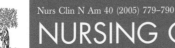

NURSING CLINICS
OF NORTH AMERICA

Integrated Primary and Mental Health Care: Evaluating a Nurse-Managed Center for Clients with Serious and Persistent Mental Illness

Judith McDevitt, PhD, APRN, BC[a],
Susan Braun, MS, APRN, BC[a],*,
Margaret Noyes, ND, APRN, BC[a],
Marsha Snyder, PhD, APRN, BC[a],
Lucy Marion, PhD, RN, FAAN[b]

[a]University of Illinois at Chicago College of Nursing, Department of Public Health, Mental Health, and Administrative Nursing, 845 South Damen Avenue, NURS (MC 802), Chicago, IL 60612, USA
[b]School of Nursing, Medical College of Georgia, 997 Saint Sebastian Way, Augusta, GA 30912, USA

N urse-managed centers have been at the forefront of providing ambulatory care alternatives for underserved populations lacking access to care [1,2]. Providing this care, however, requires reaching the population effectively, assuring informed practice management, and finding solutions to the financial dilemmas in sustaining operations. Typically, the clients served in nurse-managed centers are uninsured or are recipients of Medicaid and Medicare, with additional funding coming from grants, gifts, and in-kind support. Many nurse-managed centers have had to close because of these daunting challenges [3].

Since 1998, the Center for Integrated Health Care (IHC), an academic nurse-managed center of the College of Nursing, University of Illinois at Chicago, has delivered primary and mental health care to a unique and underserved population, clients with serious and persistent mental illness (SPMI) who are enrolled in psychosocial rehabilitation. The authors' experience illustrates the many rewards and the significant challenges that nurse-managed centers face. To evaluate progress, identify future goals, and share the authors' experience

This work was supported by the Division of Nursing, Bureau of Health Professions, Health Resources and Services Administration, US Department of Health and Human Services, Grant #D11HP00152-05-00, and The Robert Wood Johnson Foundation, Local Initiative Funding Partners Program.

*Corresponding author. E-mail address: sbraun@uic.edu (S. Braun).

0029-6465/05/$ – see front matter
doi:10.1016/j.cnur.2005.08.004

with others, this article will (1) describe their center's model of integrated care developed for its unique clientele; (2) examine selected performance indicators, including staffing, clinical services, and financing; and (3) discuss implications, opportunities, and challenges ahead.

DEVELOPING A MODEL OF INTEGRATED CARE

Health of people with serious and persistent mental illness

SPMI—such as schizophrenia, bipolar illness, or major depression—is a leading cause of disability [4]. The disability of SPMI is related not only to mental illness, but also to poor physical health. For example, people with SPMI are at higher risk than the general population for hypertension, diabetes, heart problems, and obesity [5,6] and have higher rates of chronic infections such as HIV and hepatitis C [7].

Commonly used psychiatric medications, while efficacious for mental health treatment, can place clients with SPMI at higher risk for obesity, diabetes, and hyperlipidemia [8,9]. Some medications are associated with QT interval prolongation on ECG, movement disorders, or other adverse effects [9]. The health and medication problems now are considered so significant that national consensus conferences are recommending ongoing physical health monitoring in patients receiving antipsychotic drugs [8,9].

Unfortunately, physical health problems in people with SPMI often go undiagnosed and untreated [10]. These unmet health care needs jeopardize successful mental health treatment and are associated with excess and earlier deaths [11]. In part, the poorer health of people with SPMI may be due to cognitive or behavioral factors associated with SPMI or the stigma of SPMI, any of which may make clients unwilling or unable to seek primary care or to receive routine preventive services [10]. But even when clients do want and are willing to use these services, many with SPMI lack access to primary care [12,13].

Integrated care

Because mental health programs are often the only continuing entrée into health care that people with SPMI may have, one solution now being developed is to provide essential primary care services integrated within mental health programs, making them more accessible [14]. This service delivery model can facilitate coordination of comprehensive, high-quality care, reduce medical comorbidities, and prevent excess and earlier deaths [15,16].

Four service delivery models of integrated care recently were studied by the Bazelon Center for Mental Health Law, Washington, DC [15]:

1. Primary care embedded in a program for people with SPMI
2. Unified primary and mental health programs
3. Mental health professionals located in a primary care setting
4. Collaboration between separate mental health and primary care practices.

The authors' nurse-managed IHC fits the first model. Integrated care is the result of primary care services being provided by nurses on site in a psychiatric rehabilitation program [17,18].

The authors' model of integrated care, however, goes beyond just providing primary care on site. Because providers are both primary care and mental health advanced practice nurses, the center's vision is to address together the primary and mental health needs of clients, thereby integrating the care itself. The IHC aims to:

- Integrate concepts, approaches, and processes of mental health nursing into the everyday provision of primary care, particularly those related to therapeutic alliance building and cognitive–behavioral change
- Expand the everyday provision of mental health nursing to incorporate concepts, approaches, and processes of primary care

Based on the Interaction Model of Client Health Behavior [19], the premise of this model is that use of care, adherence to recommended care, and health status will improve when nurses effectively tailor care by providing appropriate health information, responding to each client's affective concerns, and engaging each client's decisional control over health behaviors.

For clients with SPMI, the authors believe that integrating mental health with primary care nursing is the best foundation for effectively tailoring care. The following are examples from the authors' practice:

- A client being seen by the family nurse practitioner (FNP) for her annual breast examination has a phobia about being touched. The FNP enlists the expertise of the psychiatric clinical nurse specialist (PCNS) to support the client while she is being examined. As a result, the breast exam is completed without anxiety on the part of the client. In fact, the client is able to learn breast self-exam and gives a return demonstration to the nurse.
- The PCNS, hearing a client report of fatigue and dizziness, consults with the FNP regarding the symptoms and makes an appropriate referral for follow-up. The PCNS gives knowledgeable attention to the client's physical symptoms and avoids erroneously attributing the symptoms to mental illness, as health care providers often do [15].
- Diabetes self-management is complex and challenging, even for people without SPMI. The cognitive and motivational deficits that often accompany mental illness further complicate effective patient education and evidence-based diabetes care. The FNP and PCNS working together developed a diabetes care flow sheet for the clinics. The flow sheet integrates tracking of the essential requirements of diabetes care with ongoing assessment of stress and lifestyle that can influence glycemic control profoundly [20].

The Center for Integrated Health Care

IHC had its inception in fall of 1997, when psychiatric nursing students in clinical rotations at a community-based mental health agency observed that many of the clients they were seeing had unmet health care needs such as rashes, dental caries, and obesity. Their instructor, Ms. Nancy Burke, consulted with colleagues at the College of Nursing to determine whether nurse practitioner faculty and students could address some of these needs.

The center opened in spring of 1998, operating one-half day per week in a single room in one of the agency's locations and providing physical exams and episodic care. Through grants from local foundations and collaboration with the agency, funds were raised to expand services and add mental health nursing. The agency remodeled space into clinics at two of their service sites, each with a reception and office area, a laboratory area, and two examination rooms. One clinic was built within the original service site, a vocational rehabilitation program for young- and middle-aged adults with SPMI, and the second clinic was built within an alternative high school for young adults with SPMI. In 2000, hours were expanded at both locations to 4 days per week. In 2002, a third clinic was opened to serve young mothers with mental illness and their babies one-half day per week, and in 2004 services were added 1 day per week at a community health center located near other program sites of the agency.

Center partnerships

Throughout the center's history, collaborations and partnerships have played a vital role. The center's community partner has been Thresholds Psychiatric Rehabilitation Centers, a large psychosocial rehabilitation agency with locations throughout metropolitan Chicago. Primary care services are provided in collaborative practice with the Department of Family Medicine, University of Illinois at Chicago. Mental health nursing services are provided in collaboration with the psychiatrist who is the medical director of Thresholds Psychiatric Rehabilitation Centers. For all visits, both for primary care and mental health services, IHC staff work closely with each client's Thresholds case manager to assure follow-up and assist with resources needed for recommended care. Other partnerships have included the Scholl College of Podiatric Medicine at Finch University, providing on-site free monthly podiatric care; and the Chicago Partnership for Health Promotion, a University of Illinois at Chicago College of Nursing program, providing ongoing nutrition education on site by a registered dietitian funded by the US Department of Agriculture.

EXAMINING PERFORMANCE INDICATORS

Central to assuring informed practice management is tracking key data over time [21]. Thresholds' staff maintains detailed, up-to-date summaries of information about their clients, including psychiatric diagnoses; age, sex, and ethnicity; and marital and employment status. From the IHC employment and billing records, staff have developed an extensive database tracking indicators such as staffing, numbers of visits, numbers of clients, characteristics of services provided, visit diagnoses, and various funded project outcomes.

For this analysis, the authors summarized Thresholds' 2004 demographic data and analyzed selected indicators from the center's most recent staffing and billing data. For staffing, numbers of visits, and numbers of clients served, the authors compared data from 2001 to 2002, 2002 to 2003, and 2003 to 2004, with subanalyses for mental health and primary care staffing. For staffing, the authors used full-time equivalencies (FTE) to facilitate comparisons with other performance analyses of nurse-managed centers. To examine trends, they calculated the number of visits per clinic day and the number of visits per client per year. As recommended by Vonderheid and colleagues [21], the authors also calculated clients, visits, and support staff level per advanced practice nurse FTE. For characteristics of services provided and visit diagnoses, they analyzed data during the most recent fiscal year, 2003 to 2004. For mental health office visits, the authors examined types of services and identified the 10 most frequent diagnoses. For primary care office visits, they examined the complexity of services (level of visit) and identified the 10 most frequent diagnoses.

Demographics
An overview of Thresholds' data provides a snapshot of the clients served by IHC. In 2004, 48% had schizophrenia; 35% had mood disorder such as bipolar disorder or major depression, and 31% had other SPMIs such as obsessive–compulsive disorder, alone or in combination with schizophrenia or mood disorder. In terms of demographics, 90% of Thresholds' members were between the ages of 20 and 59; 59% were male; 43% were white, and 50% were black. About 5% were living with a spouse or partner, while 72% were single and never married. Only 15% were fully employed, with the rest partially employed or unemployed (personal communication, Thresholds Research Department, April 28, 2005).

Staffing and clinical services
Table 1 displays data for staffing, visits, and clients for fiscal years 2001 to 2002, 2002 to 2003, and 2003 to 2004. Over 80% of the center's FTEs for all 3 years were provided by family nurse practitioners delivering primary care, with the other 16% to 18% of FTEs being psychiatric clinical nurse specialists and a psychiatric nurse practitioner providing mental health care. Reflecting the FTEs, over 80% of visits were for primary care, and the other 10% to 18% were visits for mental health care.

Although total FTEs were similar across the 3 years, the number of unduplicated clients served increased 15% in the first two years (2001 to 2002 and 2002 to 2003) and then declined slightly, from 638 in 2002 to 2003 to 622 in 2003 to 2004. During 2001 to 2002, 40% of the clients seen were new clients. The percentage of new clients declined each year thereafter, from 24.7% in 2002 to 2003 to 20.5% in 2003 to 2004. Similar to trends in clients served, total visits increased 24% from 2001 to 2002 to 2002 to 2003 but increased only 6% in the second and third years (2002 to 2003 and 2003 to 2004). From 2002 to 2003, support staff was added at each clinic site, and this contributed to increased productivity. In the following year, there were no changes in support staffing levels and little change in total visits or visits per clinic day.

Visits per client per year ranged from 6.24 to 7.33 visits across the 3 years. This is approximately twice as many visits per year as the 3.4 visits persons without SPMI make for ambulatory care each year [22] and may reflect the multiple comorbidities of the center's population. Visits per clinic day increased 24% (6.3 to 7.8 visits per day) during the first 2 years (2001 to 2002 and 2002 to 2003) and increased a lesser amount, to 8.3 visits per day, from 2003 to 2004. There was no clinical support staff from 2001 to 2002 (only administrative

Table 1
Integrated Health Care staffing and clinical services for fiscal years 2001–2002, 2002–2003, and 2003–2004

Integrated Health Care (IHC) indicator	2001–2002	2002–2003	2003–2004
Staffing (FTE)			
Mental health (%)	0.5 (17.9)	0.5 (16.1)	0.5 (18.5)
Primary care (%)	2.3 (82.1)	2.6 (83.9)	2.2 (81.5)
Total APN	2.8	3.1	2.7
Support staff	0.8	2.8	2.8
Clients served[a]			
New clients (%)	222 (40)	158 (24.8)	128 (20.6)
Established clients (%)	333 (60)	480 (75.2)	494 (79.4)
Total clients	555	638	622
Visits provided			
Mental health care (%)	351 (10.1)	687 (15.9)	662 (14.5)
Primary care (%)	3113 (89.9)	3625 (84.1)	3896 (85.5)
Total visits	3464	4312	4558
Utilization and performance indicators			
Visits per clinic day[b]	6.3	7.8	8.3
Visits per client per year[c]	6.2	6.8	7.3
Number per total APN FTE			
Support staff	0.3	0.9	1.0
Visits per year	1237.1	1390.9	1688.1
Clients per year	198.2	205.8	230.4

Abbreviations: APN, advanced practice nurse; FTE, full-time equivalent.
  Support staff is comprised of clinical (receptionist, registered nurse) and administrative (IHC director) staff.
  [a]Combines unduplicated mental health care clients and primary care clients.
  [b]Calculated at 400 days of primary care plus 125 days of mental health care provided at two clinic sites plus 50 half days of pediatric care provided at Mother-Baby program for a total of 550 clinic days.
  [c]Combines mental health visits and primary care visits.

support), but 0.6 and 0.7 clinical staff per advance practice nurse (APN) FTE was added in the following 2 years. This likely contributed to the growth in visits per year per APN FTE from 1237.1 visits in the first year (2001 to 2002) to 1688.1 visits in the third year (2003 to 2004), a 36% increase over the 3 years. Clients per year per APN FTE also increased, from 198.2 clients in the first year (2001 to 2002) to 230.4 clients in the third year (2003 to 2004), a 16% increase over the 3 years.

Visit characteristics and diagnoses

Table 2 displays visit characteristics and the top 10 diagnoses during 2003 to 2004 visits. For mental health care, individual psychotherapy visits of 20 to 30 minutes were provided most frequently, accounting for 94% of visits. Similar to Thresholds' demographics, in which 48% of the clients had a diagnosis of schizophrenia and schizo–affective disorder, 51.3% of the mental health visits were related to these same two diagnoses. Mood disorders such as bipolar disorder or depression affected 35% of the agency's clients but were cited less

Table 2
Visit characteristics and diagnoses for mental health care visits and primary care visits, Integrated Health Care fiscal year 2003–2004

Mental health care visits[a]		Primary care visits[a]	
Type of service	%	Level of visit	%
Individual psychotherapy, 20–30 min	94	Level 1	24.8
Individual psychotherapy, 45–50 min	6	Level 2	28.4
		Level 3	32.5
		Level 4	7.0
		Level 5	7.4
Top 10 mental health diagnoses		Top 10 primary care diagnoses	
Schizophrenia	29.9	Diabetes type 2	8.8
Schizoaffective disorder	21.4	Hypertension	8.7
Bipolar disorder	16.5	Obesity	8.4
Substance abuse	15.8	Medication use; high-risk/long-term	7.7
Depression	5.7	Hyperlipidemia	7.6
Generalized anxiety disorder	3.6	Tobacco abuse	6.0
Psychosis	2.3	General medical exam, adult	3.8
Conduct disorder	1.4	Tuberculosis screening	3.2
Obsessive–compulsive disorder	1.4	Immunization, one or more	2.4
Post-traumatic stress disorder	0.8	Counseling, dietary	2.1

[a]Combines new and established patients.

often in relation to mental health visits, where 22.2% of the diagnoses were for bipolar disorder or depression.

Primary care office visits classified by level of complexity indicate that low complexity level 1 and 2 visits accounted for slightly over half of all visits from 2003 to 2004, with moderate and higher complexity visits requiring greater decision making accounting for the remainder. The diagnoses cited most frequently reflect this distribution of complexity, with more straightforward provision of immunizations, dietary counseling, screening for tuberculosis, and monitoring of high-risk medication use accounting for 4 of the top 10 diagnoses cited. Four other diagnoses, however, are among the top 20 diagnoses in ambulatory care (hypertension, diabetes, general medical examination, and lipid disorders), and education regarding diet, weight reduction, and tobacco use are among the top 10 services provided in ambulatory care [22].

Financial indicators

IHC has had significant grant funding since opening in 1998, with the Alberto Culver Jump Start Foundation ($10,000), the Washington Square Foundation ($38,500), and the Visiting Nurses Association ($58,267) providing key start-up support for salaries and equipment purchases. In 1999, the College of Nursing was awarded a 5-year $1.2 million Basic Nurse Education and Practice grant by the US Department of Health and Human Services, Bureau of Health Professions, Division of Nursing (DON), to implement the IHC program. These funds were instrumental in providing the needed staff and management infrastructure as the integrated model of care was developed.

Table 3 displays revenue sources for fiscal years 2001 to 2004 and revenue projections for fiscal years 2004 to 2007. From 2001 to 2002, grant funding, primarily the DON grant, provided 80% of the center's support. Grants continued to provide significant funding, although levels declined to 64% and 44% of total funding during the following 2 years. Clients are insured primarily by Medicaid (70% of clients) and Medicare (27%). As such, insurance revenues have contributed only approximately 20% of total funding per year. Small service contracts for school nursing and medication management contribute another 2% to 3% of funding. As Table 3 indicates, in-kind contributions by both the College of Nursing and Thresholds have provided the critical margin to continue operations, rising to 28% of total funding by 2003 to 2004.

One possible avenue to increase revenue is to pursue enhanced reimbursement for Medicare and Medicaid visits, as would be available under a Bureau of Primary Health Care Federally Qualified Health Center (FQHC) designation. The projections in Table 3 for 2004 to 2007 display this possible scenario.

IMPLICATIONS, OPPORTUNITIES, AND CHALLENGES AHEAD

IHC faces substantial challenges over the next 3 years. Chief among these is financial sustainability, the linchpin of program planning [23]. The services provided must produce enough revenue that services can continue. The stark reality is no margin, no mission [23,24].

The evaluation data reviewed in this article indicate that the center's sustainability is at risk because of several factors well recognized in the literature. The population IHC serves is underinsured [21] (97% Medicaid and Medicare), so that reimbursements only account for 20% of income (see Table 3). Because most Thresholds' clients rely on Medicaid and Medicare, as is commonly the case in people with SPMI, the prospects appear unlikely for IHC to develop

Table 3
Integrated Health Care actual and projected revenue sources by percent of total funding for fiscal years 2001–2007

| | Percent of total funding by fiscal year | | | | | |
| | Actual | | | Projected | | |
	2001–2002	2002–2003	2003–2004	2004–2005	2005–2006	2006–2007
Grants	80	64	44	67	43	13
Service contracts	0	2	3	2	1	1
Gifts	1	1	6	1	1	1
In-kind*	5	13	28	14	11	11
Medicaid/Medicare						
Standard rate	14	20	19	16	8	0
FQHC rate	N/A	N/A	N/A	N/A	36	74

*In-kind contributions include direct revenue into the program for items such as salary expenses by the university and participating partners. These data do not include fully additional in-kind contributions by both partners for items such as rent and utilities.

diverse revenue sources such as private insurance reimbursements and capitated contracts [21,24–26]. Yet reliance on grant funding places IHC at risk of closure. Since the late 1970s, the US Department of Health and Human Services, Health Resources and Services Administration (HRSA) through DON, Bureau of Health Professions has funded nurse-managed centers to provide care in the community while educating students and providing practice opportunities for faculty [27]. Unfortunately, funding for these programs lasts only 5 years and, as the case of the IHC illustrates, once funding is over, nursing centers find it difficult to generate the needed revenue to keep their doors open. In fact, during the period from 1993 to 2001, 70 nursing centers were funded by HRSA, and 27 (39%) have been forced to close [28].

Community Health Centers (CHCs) and FQHCs are the nation's designated safety net providers [29]. Nurse-managed centers are similar to CHCs and FQHCs in the clients they serve [28], but the safety net they are providing is frequently invisible, leaving them to struggle on their own with reimbursement policies that limit their ability to fulfill their role [30]. For CHCs and FQHCs, the federal government's prospective payment system provides a higher level of reimbursement for Medicaid and Medicare patients, allowing them to recover 89% of costs [28]. The system also makes a capitation payment for each client with no insurance to cover the cost of uninsured care [28].

Although the IHC is too small and would face obstacles as an academic entity in becoming an FQHC itself, partnering with an FQHC could be a viable means to provide for future sustainability. In 2004, IHC partnered with a CHC affiliated with the University of Illinois at Chicago. This is the first step toward fully realizing the potential of FQHC partnership to enable most if not all of encounters to be reimbursed at FQHC rates. As was shown in the Table 3 projections, FQHC reimbursement mechanisms could provide greater than 70% of funding by fiscal year 2006 to 2007 if the necessary partnerships can be made. If successful, IHC would be on its way to financial security. Significant, positive factors operating are that Thresholds is supporting and assisting the IHC in these efforts. The center's unique mission of serving people with SPMI has attracted substantial funding over the years, including the current funding from The Robert Wood Johnson Foundation's Local Initiative Funding Partners Program. This award was made possible because Thresholds raised the required matching funds. It includes FQHC partnership among its goals.

A second area of challenges for IHC lies in improving patient volume, numbers, productivity, and efficiency. Clients with SPMI are certainly resource intensive, and this is another risk factor affecting sustainability [24]. At present, the attainable visit volume for IHC clients appears to be about one visit per hour, and the typical client is making seven visits per year (see Table 1). A more optimal patient mix would include patients needing less frequent preventive or minor episodic care [21], freeing up time for more billable visits.

The growth of the client base also warrants attention. Trends in the total number of clients, the number of new clients, the total number of visits, and visits per clinic day may indicate that the IHC clinic sites were reaching capacity by 2003 to 2004 given staffing levels, practice efficiencies, patient use patterns, and marketing outreach. As Table 1 indicates, volume was stabilizing at about 4500 visits, 600 clients, and a declining percentage of new clients each year. A significant expansion is underway with the "Doorway to Integrated Health Care" initiative funded by The Robert Wood Johnson Foundation's Local Initiative Funding Partners Program. The main goal of this award is to offer services to all clients of Thresholds from 2004 to 2007, thus expanding IHC's client base and generating more visits.

The visits per client per year (see Table 1) may indicate inappropriate use of care, reflecting the ready accessibility of the IHC clinics within psychosocial treatment programs. Mental health services, however, typically involve multiple visits, as does continuing care of chronic conditions such as hypertension, hyperlipidemia, or diabetes. Because cognitive and motivational deficits typically accompany SMPI, a higher number of visits per client may be needed to manage health goals appropriately. These differing explanations indicate an area for research in the future.

Compared with nurse-managed centers in the Michigan Academic Consortium (MAC) [21], IHC performance indicators (see Table 1) are on the low end of reported ranges. For support staff per APN FTE, the IHC range was 0.3 to 1.0, and the MAC range was 0.65 to 2.48, indicating higher levels of support staff for MAC. For visits per year per APN FTE, the IHC range was 1237.1 to 1688.1, and the MAC range was 1088 to 3917, indicating more visits per APN per year for MAC. For clients per year per APN FTE, the IHC range was 198.2 to 230.4, and the MAC range was 252 to 1479, indicating that MAC APNs had larger panels of patients. None of the MAC centers served clients with SPMI, so these differences may reflect the resource-intensive nature of IHC's practice.

The levels of visits and most frequent primary care diagnoses (see Table 2) indicate areas in which efficiencies could be gained. From 2003 to 2004, level 1 visits comprised almost 25% of visits, and these are visits that could be provided by a registered nurse or assistant rather than an APN. Similarly, in that 4 of the 10 most frequent diagnoses were for straightforward problems such as tuberculosis screening, reconfiguration of clinical staff to provide such services could optimize productivity of APNs to provide more level 3 and 4 visits for higher reimbursements [24]. Increased attention could also be given to appropriate coding of visits to properly reflect the complexities of caring for clients with SPMI and maximize receivables [21,25].

The third area of challenges relates to the IHC mission and model of care. Although it is clear that ensuring sustainability, growing productivity, and increasing efficiencies are vital priorities, providing primary care for people with SPMI is different than it is for people without SPMI. It involves a different set of approaches and competencies the authors believe IHC is uniquely prepared to identify, develop, and disseminate in concert with its community partner. This is the promise of IHC's model of integrated care, and the challenge is to preserve and grow the model while working on performance and sustainability. Thus in pursuing an FQHC affiliation, the authors believe that it is essential the IHC's voice as a nurse-managed center and that of its community partner be assured. As part of an FQHC affiliation, participation in the oversight of care in addition to providing the care itself would afford ongoing opportunities to further operationalize and rationalize IHC's model of care in the context of a new, three-way partnership between IHC, Thresholds, and an FQHC. If successful, this would provide lasting benefits for IHC clients and others in mental health treatment programs, and it would have applications for behavioral health programs in primary care generally.

This evaluation provides a beginning appraisal of the accomplishments and prospects for IHC's unique model of care. For evaluation to be comprehensive, further analysis is needed of costs and quality and outcomes of care [3,24,25,31,32]. Because providing care for people who have SPMI may have different costs, quality indicators, and outcomes than care in other populations, these evaluations will be important contributions to understanding whether mental health treatment can be improved by providing integrated care and how it can be provided best.

Many people living with SPMI lack access to primary care [12]. By embedding primary care services within a mental health program, individuals with SPMI are able to directly access primary care [15]. The authors believe their model of integrated care will help deliver improved health outcomes for clients with SPMI. If the financial sustainability of IHC can be secured through an FQHC affiliation, developing and testing the model and demonstrating its outcomes though well-designed clinical research will be among the challenges ahead for advancing knowledge about integrated care.

References

[1] Turkeltaub M. Nurse-managed centers: increasing access to care. J Nurs Educ 2004;43(2): 53–4.

[2] Lundeen SP. An alternative paradigm for promoting health in communities. Fam Community Health 1999;21:15–28.

[3] Vincent D, Oakley D, Pohl J, et al. Survival of nurse-managed centers: the importance of cost analysis. Outcomes Manag Nurs Pract 2000;4(3):124–8.

[4] National Institute of Mental Health. The numbers count: mental disorders in America. A summary of statistics describing the prevalence of mental disorders in America. Available at: http://www.nimh.nih.gov/publicat/numbers.cfm. Accessed March 4, 2005.

[5] Davidson S, Judd F, Jolley D, et al. Cardiovascular risk factors for people with mental illness. Aust N Z J Psychiatry 2001;35:196–202.

[6] Dixon L, Postrado L, Delahanty J, et al. The association of medical comorbidity in schizophrenia with poor physical and mental health. J Nerv Ment Dis 1999;187:496–502.

[7] Rosenberg SD, Goodman LA, Osher FC, et al. Prevalence of HIV, hepatitis B, and hepatitis C in people with severe mental illness. Am J Public Health 2001;91:31–7.

[8] American Diabetes Association, American Psychiatric Association, American Association of Clinical Endocrinologists, and North American Association for the Study of Obesity. Consensus development conference on antipsychotic drugs and obesity and diabetes. Diabetes Care 2004;27(2):596–601.

[9] Marder SR, Essock SM, Miller AL, et al. Physical health monitoring of patients with schizophrenia. Am J Psychiatry 2004;161(8):1334–49.

[10] Felker B, Yazel JJ, Short D. Mortality and medical comorbidity among psychiatric patients: a review. Psychiatr Serv 1996;47:1356–63.

[11] Brown S. Excess mortality of schizophrenia: a meta-analysis. Br J Psychiatry 1997;171: 502–8.

[12] Druss BG, Rosenheck RA. Mental disorders and access to medical care in the United States. Am J Psychiatry 1998;155:1775–7.

[13] Miller CL, Druss BG, Dombrowski EA, et al. Barriers to primary medical care among patients at a community mental health center. Psychiatr Serv 2003;54(8):1158–60.

[14] Druss BG, Rohrbaugh RM, Levinson CM, et al. Integrated medical care for patients with serious mental illness: a randomized trial. Arch Gen Psychiatry 2001;58(9):861–8.

[15] Koyanagi C. Get it together: how to integrate physical and mental health care for people with serious mental disorders. Washington (DC): Bazelon Center for Mental Health Law; 2004.

[16] US Department of Health and Human Services. Report of a Surgeon Generals' working meeting on the integration of mental health services and primary health care. Available at: http://www.surgeongeneral.gov/library/mentalhealthservices/mentalhealthservices. html. Accessed April 6, 2005.

[17 Marion LN, Braun S, Anderson D, et al. Center for integrated health care: primary and mental health care for people with severe and persistent mental illness. J Nurs Educ 2004;43(2): 71–4.

[18] McDevitt J, Rose DN, Marion L. Integrating primary and mental health care in an innovative educational model. Nurs Health Care Perspect 2002;22(2):62–3.

[19] Cox CL. An interaction model of client health behavior: theoretical prescription for nursing. ANS Adv Nurs Sci 1982;5:541–56.

[20] McDevitt J, Synder M, Breitmayer B, et al. Diabetes management in the context of serious and persistent mental illness: clinical practice recommendations for integrated care. Available at: http://www.uic.edu/nursing/pma/services/diabetes/research/index.htm. Accessed May 9, 2005.

[21] Vonderheid S, Pohl J, Shafer P, et al. Using FTE and RVU performance measures to assess financial viability of academic nurse-managed centers. Nurs Econ 2004;22(3): 124–34.

[22] Woodwell DA, Cherry DK. National ambulatory medical care survey: 2002 summary. Advance data from vital and health statistics; no 346. Hyattsville (MD): National Center for Health Statistics; 2004.

[23] Esperat MC, Green A, Acton C. One vision of academic nursing centers. Nurs Econ 2004;22(6):307–19.

[24] Vonderheid S, Pohl J, Barkauskas V, et al. Financial performance of nurse-managed primary care centers. Nurs Econ 2003;21(4):167–75.

[25] Barkauskas VH, Pohl J, Breer L, et al. Academic nurse-managed centers: approaches to evaluation. Outcomes Manag 2004;8(1):57–66.

[26] Swan BA, Cotroneo M. Financing strategies for a community nursing center. Nurs Econ 1999;17(1):44–8.

[27] Barger S. Academic nursing centers: the road from the past, the bridge to the future. J Nurs Educ 2004;43(2):60–5.

[28] National Nursing Center Consortium. Congressional briefing. March 18, 2005: Nurse-managed health centers: an emerging safety-net provider. 2005. Available at: http://www.nncc.us/policy/policy.html. Accessed April 23, 2005.

[29] Lewin ME, Altman S. America's health care safety net: intact but endangered (executive summary). Washington (DC): National Science Foundation, IOM; 2000.

[30] Pohl JM, Vonderheid SC, Barkauskas VH, et al. The safety net: academic nurse-managed centers' role. Policy, Politics & Nursing Practice 2004;5(2):84–94.

[31] Ervin NE, Chang WY, White J. A cost analysis of a nursing center's services. Nurs Econ 1998;16(6):307–12.

[32] Hunter JK, Ventura MR, Kearns PA. Cost analysis of a nursing center for the homeless. Nurs Econ 1999;17(1):20–8.

Nurs Clin N Am 40 (2005) 791–801

NURSING CLINICS
OF NORTH AMERICA

ELSEVIER
SAUNDERS

A Health Care Program for Homeless Children Using Healthy People 2010 Objectives

Yvonne Yousey, RN, CPNP, PhD[a],*, Michelle Carr, RN, BSN[b]

[a]Department of Family and Community Nursing, University of North Carolina at Charlotte, 9201 University City Boulevard, Charlotte, NC 28223, USA
[b]University of North Carolina Nursing Center for Health Promotion, 534 Spratt Street, Charlotte, NC 28206, USA

C hildren in homeless shelters have urgent and chronic health needs, with limited access to health care services. A health care program based on Healthy People 2010 objectives provides screening and treatment to these children through a nursing center in a homeless shelter. The nursing center provides service using intervention protocols based on levels of prevention and national standards for care; outcomes of interventions are measured and recorded through a software tracking system. Education modules in nutrition, oral, and dental care focus on primary prevention; secondary prevention includes lead, hearing, vision, and mental health screening, and assessment of environmental tobacco smoke exposure. Health problems, identified through physical assessment, are treated or referred for further follow-up, and chronic problems are managed in collaboration with community agencies. Outcome measures provide information regarding the ability of the child health program to meet health needs of homeless children who have no regular source of health care or who are unable to use this care.

Aggressive screening, effective treatment of health problems, and preventive health care offer the possibility of improving the health status and well-being of homeless children through a nursing clinic at a homeless shelter [1]. Children who are homeless have adverse health consequences because of their complex health problems, and health care systems are limited in their ability to address the health and social needs of these children and their families [1]. A comprehensive child health program, using Healthy People 2010 objectives, national standards of health care, clinical guidelines, and policy recommendations by American Academy of Pediatrics (AAP) and American Academy of Family Practice, is being implemented to target the unique needs of these children. The program includes screening, anticipatory guidance, case management, transitional

*Corresponding author. E-mail address: ykyousey@uncc.edu (Y. Yousey).

0029-6465/05/$ – see front matter
doi:10.1016/j.cnur.2005.08.003

primary care, and health education. Collaboration with community agencies provides a range of services, not possible with limited staff at the nursing center. Outcome measures monitor the implementation and effects of these partners in the health program. This program was developed to evaluate the health outcomes of children who have access to a health care program through a homeless shelter.

BACKGROUND

Addressing health issues of families who are homeless is complicated by health and social issues. Families with children comprise approximately 40% of 1 to 2 million homeless individuals on any given night [2]. Fifty percent of homeless persons are African American; 35% are white; 12% are Hispanic, and 2% are Native American [3]. Families with children, the fastest growing segment, account for up to 43% of the homeless population [4], a result of the trend to de-institutionalize persons with mental illnesses and changes in social service policies over the past two decades [1,5].

The rate of increasing homelessness has resulted in poor health outcomes for children. Most are eligible for Medicaid, but the chaos and complex social issues in their lives preclude many from using the services as intended. Homeless children are more likely to use emergency rooms for health care needs and are less likely to receive preventive care from a regular provider [6]. They receive sporadic health care because of the lack of transportation, inability to maneuver through the health care system, and the competing demands for food and shelter [6]. Other barriers include the denial of their health problems by their parents, and health care providers' misconceptions, prejudices, and frustrations in dealing with the issues associated with homelessness [1].

Children who are homeless are more likely to come from backgrounds of domestic violence and abuse, placing them at greater risk for mental health problems, psychiatric morbidity, and exposure to environmental conditions exacerbating illness [5]. These conditions lead to a wide range of other health problems including poor hygiene, nutritional deficiencies, trauma, exposure, accidents, victimization, and infections [7]. Delays in routine screening and immunizations, high rates of acute and chronic illness, dental problems, lack of access to primary care, and increased use of emergency rooms and hospitalizations are common problems [6]. They also suffer from failure to thrive and physical problems such as respiratory, ear, and skin infections. Illnesses such as anemia, asthma, and recurrent otitis media go undiagnosed and untreated. Infectious diseases are common because of the potential for rapid spread among people living in crowded shelters [7].

The effects of homelessness on normal childhood development include academic difficulty, behavior problems, growth delay, anxiety, depression, and learning difficulties [7]. Greater incidence of developmental delays, behavior problems, and poor academic performance has been documented in children who are homeless compared with housed counterparts [5]. Delays in areas of cognitive ability, language development, motor skills, and social interaction place them at risk for academic failure [8].

Community health programs have provided on-site services that address access-to-care issues for homeless women and their children. Berti and colleagues [5] reported on the effectiveness of school-based health centers in meeting the health needs of homeless children. Academic settings provide limited services through medical and nursing students [9]. In the community in which the nursing center is located, only one small program addresses needs of homeless children and limits its scope of services to referral and case management. Most programs have not developed strategies that address the challenging demands of homeless children. Services lack sources of funding, and no consistent approaches in screening exist to identify health issues and treatment options for families. To date, there are no outcome measures associated with programs that target homeless women and children, in spite of the increase and complexity of health problems in this population.

IMPLEMENTING A PROGRAM FOR CHILDREN WHO ARE HOMELESS

A nurse-managed center, located on site at a homeless shelter, uses a model of community-based health care delivery, providing health education, comprehensive health screening, transitional care for chronic illnesses, and case management and referral services for women and children. Community health nurses in the center provide nonprescription medications through a self-help station, prescription assistance, individual health teaching and health education classes, developmental screening, anticipatory guidance, case management, and referral. In addition, nurse practitioners provide episodic care for those with minor acute illnesses and transitional care for those with chronic illnesses. This nursing center has been providing services for 10 years and serves as a site for faculty practice and service learning for undergraduate and graduate nursing students enrolled in the university. Presently, over 6000 health care visits are provided each year.

Strategies for provision of care at the nursing center consider the unique characteristics of homeless families. Because of their social isolation, most homeless persons do not trust care providers or institutions [9]. Their disaffiliation creates a need for community outreach and the development of a trusting relationship between health care providers and the residents of the homeless shelter. The nursing center strengthens trust by offering services on site. Levy and O'Connell suggest that cost-effective primary and preventive care for homeless people is possible if providers are willing to provide personalized, individualized care directly to the streets and shelters [9]. The concern for the next meal and the night's shelter are far more pressing than health care needs. The nursing center is open during hours that clients can most easily use it, from 3 p.m. to 7 p.m. each weeknight. An open-door policy welcomes clients into the nursing center during these hours. Appointments are encouraged but not necessary. Clients are assisted with transportation to health care facilities for services. Case management services help residents apply for Medicaid or other assistance. The community health nurse also assists residents who have

Medicaid to find a primary care provider. Transportation is provided for people who need emergent care. Coordination with on-site social workers provides other services needed by families.

Child health interventions involving education and anticipatory guidance are based on *Bright Futures: Guidelines for Health Supervision of Infants, Children, and Adolescents,* national guidelines for well-child care [10]. Group and individual educational sessions are organized into modules and provide information on topics selected from Healthy People 2010 objectives. (Table 1). Outcomes that will be measured include pre- or post-testing for parent knowledge, number of problems identified through screening, number of referrals, use of tools to evaluate mental health status, and referrals.

PROGRAM IMPLEMENTATION

Healthy People 2010 objectives present a comprehensive, nationwide health promotion and disease prevention agenda to eliminate health disparities [11]. These objectives provided the guiding framework for the program targeting children served by the nursing center who suffer increased morbidity and mortality related to poverty and the lack of permanent shelter. Protocols for screening, education, and referral were developed based on AAP [13] and Bright Futures guidelines [10]. Specific age-appropriate actions and interventions were developed using levels of prevention framework. Evidenced-based guidelines following national standards for management of chronic illnesses were used in providing transitional care for chronic illnesses such as anemia and asthma. Measurement outcomes for each objective were identified, and a data collection system was established using a software program. Collaborative agreements were established with other community agencies to provide health education services already available in the community. Health outcomes of individual children are measured by looking at change of health status, functioning, quality of life, self-management of disease, client choice in care, and client satisfaction [7]. This program was approved by the Human Subjects Interdisciplinary Board at University of North Carolina, Charlotte.

The child health program in this nursing center was developed to provide a consistent, cost-effective approach in addressing health issues of children residing in the shelter. Specific screening activities and assessment identify risks and problems associated with mental health, nutrition, oral and dental health, developmental delays, exposure to violence and abuse, and access to primary care [11]. Various strategies including group education, individual counseling, and hand-outs provide health education and information on these topics.

A pediatric nurse practitioner provides comprehensive physical assessment of children. Children are identified when they come to the shelter and are brought to the nursing center, where they receive a complete physical exam and age-appropriate screening for health risks. The nurse practitioner and community health nurse screen for nutrition and oral health problems, mental health, tobacco smoke exposure, and vision, hearing, development, and lead exposure using history and valid, reliable tools if available. Once

Table 1
Summary of Healthy People 2010 Objectives—child health program

Health People 2010 objectives	Goals based on objectives	Age groups targeted	Measures of outcomes
Access to care	Increase number with health insurance. Increase number with primary care provider. Reduce difficulties, delays in obtaining care.	All	Number counseled
Nutrition	Reduce overweight, obesity	All	Number of education sessions, number of referrals
	Increase intake of fruits, vegetables. Reduce intake of sodium, fat. Reduce iron deficiency anemia. Reduce hunger.		
Oral health	Reduce untreated dental decay Increase regular, preventive dental visits.	All	Number counseled, number of referrals
Physical activity	Increase physical activity in adolescents.	Adolescents	Number counseled
Tobacco smoke exposure and substance abuse	Reduce tobacco initiation and use among adolescents. Increase smoking cessation counseling. Reduce tobacco smoke exposure. Increase treatment for substance use.	Adolescents	Number counseled, number of referrals
Psychosocial/ mental health issues	Increase screening for identification of mental health issues and treatment for identified problems.	Preschoolers through adolescents	Number identified, number of referrals
Growth and development— safety	Increase number of children using car seats and vehicle restraints.	All	Number counseled
	Increase number of infants sleeping on backs.	Infants	
Hearing and vision	Decrease number of uncorrected visual problems.	Preschoolers, school-age, adolescents	Number identified, number of referrals
	Increase number of hearing/ vision screening tests.		

risks are identified, anticipatory guidance and education are provided either individually or in groups. Health problems are treated on site or referred to appropriate resources. Funding through a local agency provides incentives to parents and children when they complete the health assessment, screening, and education.

The nutrition program focuses on identifying nutritional deficits in children. Nutritional status is assessed by history, growth parameters (height, weight, and body mass index [BMI]), and hemoglobin. The nurse practitioner assesses eating behaviors, need for fluoride supplementation, and evaluates the appearance of the child's skin, hair, teeth, and gums. Information on age-appropriate feeding techniques and foods is provided based on guidelines outlined in *Bright Futures in Practice: Nutrition* [13]. Children's growth is assessed by height, weight, and BMI. Children are considered to be at risk for obesity if they have a BMI of 85% or greater for age. Children whose height and weight are less than the 3% for age are referred to a primary care provider for continued follow-up. Vitamins and iron supplementation are provided to children who have been identified with anemia. Referrals to the local Women, Infants, and Children (WIC) program are made for age-appropriate children. Other children who are identified as needing more work-up are referred.

A second component of the nutrition program involves a nutrition education program for shelter meal providers. A registered dietician works with the staff to provide nutritious, healthy meals for the residents. Observation of meals offered in the dining room before and after the education sessions will be used to evaluate the program. The community health nurse provides four nutrition education programs at regular times in the nursing center, each lasting approximately 20 minutes. These programs were developed by a registered dietician and include topics such as: healthy meals, healthy snacks, beverages, and building strong bones and muscles. Learning is measured before and after programs. Mothers and their children attend individually or in groups and receive healthy snacks at the completion of each session.

Dental problems are assessed at the time of physical assessment. Dental health is assessed through history and examination of child's teeth for malocclusion or cavities [14]. The nurse practitioner obtains information on oral care and habits through a dental screening form that provides information on dental visits and oral hygiene practices in the family. Each child receives a cursory dental examination during the physical examination. Education on oral care is provided using guidelines in *Bright Futures in Health: Oral Health* [14]. Dental visits are recommended based on guidelines established by AAP and American Dental Association for routine dental care [12]. Referrals are made immediately for children who have cavities or other oral health problems, and assistance is provided to families to access the care. A dental education program developed by a grant-funded community agency is provided once monthly for women and their children. At this session, they receive information and education on nutrition that promote healthy teeth, proper care of teeth at various ages, and information on where to find dental care.

Development is assessed using the Denver II developmental screening tool in children, newborn to age 6. Anticipatory guidance and education on various aspects of growth and development are provided. When children are identified as being at risk, a physical exam is done to rule out other findings. Interventions for increased stimulation are provided to parents, and the child is re-checked. If the child does not make progress, referral for further work-up is done.

Hearing and vision screening are completed on all children over age 3. Vision is assessed through history and by Snellen test, and hearing is evaluated using audiometry. When children with potential problems are identified, a physical exam is done to confirm findings, and children are referred for further diagnostic testing and treatment.

Lead screening is done based on guidelines from the AAP [12]. A questionnaire assesses risk for lead exposure. Blood lead levels are drawn for any children who have identified risk factors such as living in an older home with chipping paint, a sibling or friend who has been treated for elevated lead levels, and living near a smelter. If elevated, children are referred for further treatment.

Immunization status is assessed based on availability of immunization records and referrals made for administration of immunizations through the local health department. No immunizations are given on site because of a collaborative agreement with the local health department.

Children are assessed for risk of environmental tobacco smoke exposure with a questionnaire inquiring about smoke exposure and smoking practices in the home. All parents are given information on protecting their children from smoke exposure. In addition, parents who smoke are given information on smoking cessation classes as requested.

The Pediatric Symptom Checklist is a psychosocial screening tool designed to recognize cognitive, emotional, and behavioral problems in children [15]. Chronic mental illness is prevalent in women (30% to 48%) who are homeless, and their children are at higher risk for developing problems [7]. The checklist is administered to mothers of children age 4 and older by the nurse practitioner. Children who have a positive score are referred for further follow-up. Mothers with identified mental health issues are followed in collaboration with behavioral health services.

Collaborative agreements with other community agencies provide education services not otherwise available to families. Dental and asthma education is provided through community agencies that come on site at appointed times. Asthma education is provided individually and is enhanced with computer activities for those able to use the computer. In addition to providing as many services as possible on site, assistance is provided when referrals and specialist visits are needed. The multiple, complex needs of families and children on the margins of existing community networks cannot be met by a single agency, or by expansion of specialty services, but through collaboration and cooperation between agencies responsible for care [7]. The nursing center and the social work staff at the homeless shelter are a vital link to the safety net of health care services for shelter residents. They provide client advocacy and collaborate with other health care agencies to access services for clients.

Homeless people respond best to provision of resources rather than educational materials to facilitate changes in behavior to increase their health [7]. Educational materials have been developed at a third to fifth grade reading level for those clients who desire them. They are used minimally, however. Instead, clients are engaged one-to-one with a staff person, at which time they may ask questions and receive information. Activities that involve one-to-one personal or group interaction are successful with these clients related to their need for meaningful human contact [7].

The emphasis on access to care in Healthy People 2010 Objectives is the basis for strategies to help shelter residents access needed services. Many families residing at the shelter leave their homes in haste, sometimes from far away, and have little or no resources. Social workers at the shelter, in collaboration with the community health nurse, assist them in applying for Medicaid and accessing other resources. If emergent medical care is needed, transportation is provided, and a referral is sent with the patient following the initial assessment at the nursing center. The community health nurse and the social workers assist families in finding a primary health care provider for ongoing health care.

EVALUATION OF HEALTH OUTCOMES

The Health Care for Homeless Branch of the Division of Special Populations/ Bureau of Primary Health Care identifies client outcomes of improved health status, functioning, and quality of life; involvement in treatment; self-management of disease; and client satisfaction as important when evaluating health care in this population [16]. Outcomes for this child health program focus on improved health status and are measured by the number of health problems identified in children, the number of referrals made, and follow-up of the referrals. Educational programs are designed to increase self-management in families and are evaluated through pre- and post testing of knowledge. Evaluation of behavior change is a more desirable outcome but not a realistic expectation in this transient population. The use of these markers will enable nurses to improve health status and assist in disease management of women and their children.

The program was initiated in January 2005, and preliminary data are now being compiled. In the first 4 months, 84 children between ages of newborn and 17 years were evaluated for either sick care or physicals; 33 children received comprehensive physical exams, and 51 children received care for minor acute illnesses. Twenty-four (72%) children were age newborn to 4 years' five (15%) were age 5 to 8 years; one (3%) was 9 to 11 years, and three (9%) were 12 to 18 years of age. Eighty screening tests in nine areas were completed on 28 children with abnormal results detected on 20 screening tests. (Table 2) All children screened for anemia had low hemoglobin findings consistent with mild or moderate iron deficiency anemia. Thirty percent of children evaluated for

Table 2
Screening tests on children

Area screened	Number of screenings	Number of abnormal screenings needing referral
Hearing	3	1 (30%)
Vision	5	5 (100%)
Height/weight/BMI	21	0
Hemoglobin for anemia	8	8 (100%)
Development	11	3 (33%)
Lead screening	7	1 (14%)
Smoke exposure	9	0
Dental	9	3 (30%)
Physical activity	7	0

dental problems were identified as having dental caries and referred for further care. All other children were referred for preventive dental care. No data are available on referrals or results of referrals.

In children seen for sick care, 115 diagnoses were associated with upper respiratory problems; 16 diagnoses were associated with gastrointestinal disturbances, and 18 were associated with skin disorders. Five diagnoses were associated with mental or psychosocial disorders. These categories are consistent with findings previously identified that indicate the types of health problems these children encounter. No data were available as to how many diagnoses each child had.

IMPLICATIONS FOR NURSING PRACTICE

The use of nurses and nurse practitioners to identify health problems, provide health education, and complete case management for high-risk families living in a homeless shelter is a cost effective method of providing care. Provision of services on site and in collaboration with community agencies to provide various health services that would not be possible otherwise further ensure that children with high risks and problems receive the services that they need. Individual- and group-focused education rarely has been used with this population but ensures a greater emphasis on prevention. To date, no programs have been able to demonstrate the efficacy of health screening or prevention efforts with families who lack housing.

Providing services to children of women who are homeless is resource intensive. Families need assistance with all aspects of care including accessing Medicaid, finding appropriate care sources for continued care follow-up, making appointments, and transportation to the appointments. These tasks are in addition to the myriad of other problems facing them. Families vary in their ability to seek out care, depending on their familiarity with the health care community and their knowledge of working through the system. The community health nurse assists the family in using whatever skills they have and supplements them to obtain the needed care.

In spite of the progress that has been made, challenges abound. The continued quest for funding to support the services needed is time consuming and never ending. Not all aspects of care are available at the shelter, even preventive services. Immunizations and screening for tuberculosis are not offered, even though this population is known to have lower immunization rates and be at greater risk for tuberculosis [7]. Changes in administration of the agency and the demands of children and families with health problems complicated by social issues make continuing these services a challenge.

Outcomes have been identified that will assist in evaluating value of services provided to families residing at the homeless shelter. As with many problems associated with homelessness, the final outcomes will not be realized during the client's stay at the shelter. Attempts to quantify any increases in health status are limited by the nature of homelessness and the health conditions that accompany it. As is true in most chronic illnesses where regression and relapse are a part of the process, the changes occurring in these families cannot be measured in a linear fashion. Instead, it will need to be done incrementally and involve an assessment matrix that considers the complexity of finances, social supports, and other psychosocial issues in addition to the health and treatment indicators that are much easier to measure [7].

This program is built on the strong foundation of health objectives that attempt to address disparities in vulnerable populations. It uses evidence-based protocols and guidelines that emulate best practices. The ability of the program to address the specific and unique needs of children in a homeless shelter and demonstrate its effectiveness through measurement of outcomes will ensure its longevity.

References

[1] Donohue M. Homelessness in the United States: history, epidemiology, health issues, women, and public policy. Available at: http://www.medscape.com. Accessed March 19, 2005.

[2] US Conference of Mayors. Sodexho hunger and homelessness survey 2003. Available at: http://usmayors.org/uscm.news/press_releases/documents/hunger_121803.asp. Accessed April 3, 2005.

[3] National Coalition for the Homeless. Education of homeless youth. 1999. Washington, DC, National Coalition for the Homeless, NCH Fact Sheet #10.

[4] American Academy of Pediatrics. Committee on Community Health Services. Health needs of homeless children and families. Pediatrics 1996;98(4):789–91.

[5] Berti L, Zylbert S, Rolnitzky L. Comparison of health status of children using a school-based health center for comprehensive care. J Pediatr Health Care 2001;15:244–50.

[6] Weinrub L, Goldberg R, Bassuk E, et al. Determinants of health and service use patterns in homeless and low-income housed children. Pediatrics 1998;102(3):554–62.

[7] McMurray-Avila M, Gelberg L, Breakey W. Balancing act: clinical practices that respond to the needs of homeless people. Presented at the 1998 National Symposium on Homelessness Research. Arlington, VA; October 29–30, 1998. Available at: http://www.aspe.hhs.gov/homeless/symposium. Accessed April 3, 2005.

[8] Morris R, Butt R. Parents' perspectives on homelessness and its effects on the education development of their children. J Sch Nurs 2003;19(1):43–50.

[9] Levy B, O'Connell J. Health care for homeless persons. N Engl J Med 2004;350(23): 2329–32.

[10] Green M, Palfrey J. (2002). Bright futures: guidelines for health supervision of infants, children, and adolescents. 2nd edition. Arlington (VA): National Center for Education in Maternal and Child Health, Georgetown University; 2002.

[11] US Department of Health and Human Services. Healthy people 2010: understanding and improving health. 2nd edition. Washington (DC): US Government Printing Office; 2000.

[12] American Academy of Pediatrics. Clinical practice guidelines and policies. 4th edition. Elk Grove Village, (IL): American Academy of Pediatrics; 2004.

[13] Story M, Holt K, Sofka D. Bright futures in practice: nutrition. 2nd edition. Arlington (VA): National Center for Education in Maternal and Child Health, Georgetown University; 2002.

[14] US Department of Health and Human Services. Bright futures in practice: oral health. Arlington (VA): National Center for Education in Maternal and Child Health, Georgetown University; 2002.

[15] Jellnick MS, Murphy JM, Little M, et al. Use of pediatric symptom checklist (PSC) to screen for psychosocial problems in pediatric primary care: a national feasibility study. Arch Pediatr Adolesc Med 1999;153(3):254–60.

[16] National Research Council and Institute of Medicine. Children's health, the nation's health: assessing and improving children's health. Washington (DC): The National Academies Press; 2002.

Nurs Clin N Am 40 (2005) 803–815

NURSING CLINICS
OF NORTH AMERICA

ELSEVIER
SAUNDERS

"My Nurse Taught Me How to Have a Healthy Baby and Be a Good Mother:" Nurse Home Visiting with Pregnant Women 1888 to 2005

Katy Dawley, PhD, CNM[a],*, Rita Beam, RN, MSN[b]

[a]Drexel University College of Nursing and Health Professions, 235 Pelham Road, Philadelphia, PA 19119, USA
[b]National Nurse Family Partnership, 1900 Grant Street, Denver, CO 80203, USA

Catherine was a frightened, unmarried, pregnant young woman in 1991 when her Nurse Family Partnership (NFP) nurse first visited her home in Elmira, New York. She did well during pregnancy. She learned about her body and how to have a healthy baby. She talked with her nurse about her life and her dreams for the future. She learned how to take baby steps toward achieving her heart's desires. Having earned a nursing degree, she now enjoys her nursing career and has gotten married. For 2 years she inspired other young women as a nurse home visitor in the same NFP program that was so important to her when faced with the life crisis of being young and pregnant too soon. Her adolescent son also benefited from his mother's experience with the NFP. He presents himself as a well-adjusted young man who already expresses his life goals.

Rebecca is a young mother living in a shelter and will graduate from the NFP in 4 months when her daughter turns 2. After spending more than 2 years in the program, she formed a very strong bond with Carol, her NFP nurse. At a visit several months before the baby's second birthday when Carol mentioned that they would be saying good-by soon, Rebecca said, "Don't tell me that, you can still teach me things" [1]. Like thousands of women since the late 1800s, Catherine and Rebecca have benefited from nurse home visits during pregnancy, in the postpartum period, and in the early years of parenting.

NURSE HOME VISITING 1888 TO 1930

Nurse home visiting with pregnant women has its origins in the late nineteenth century when neither physicians nor midwives scheduled regular prenatal visits. Regular prenatal visits first occurred when visiting nurses in Philadelphia

*Corresponding author. E-mail address: kd25@drexel.edu (K. Dawley).

started making biweekly home visits with pregnant women. The impetus was the discovery of a very ill and unsupervised boy at home by a nurse from the Visiting Nurses Association (VNA). His term pregnant mother was an in-patient in Preston Maternity Hospital, and his father worked long hours away from home to support the family. Medical efforts to help him were unsuccessful, and he died of his illness [2]. The problem identified by the VNA nurses was that Preston Maternity Hospital, in an effort prevent puerperal fever, hospitalized women during the last month of pregnancy in an effort to improve their nutrition and eliminate infection. After delivery, they kept new mothers in the hospital for the first month postpartum, thus placing other children at similar risk.

The Philadelphia VNA's solution was to institute a nurse home visiting program for pregnant women to improve health throughout pregnancy to decrease these extended hospital stays. Nurse visits were the first periodic health care provided to women during pregnancy, and within a few years, prenatal visits comprised a large percentage of the VNA's workload [2]. In 1901, the second prenatal visiting nurse service began at the Instructive District Nursing Association of Boston. Following the success of these services, nurses at VNAs throughout the country and at nurse-managed organizations, such as Henry Street Settlement and Maternity Center Association in New York, visited pregnant women and made postpartum visits. The content of these visits modeled what later became routine prenatal care.

Visiting nurses provided education with the intention of improving birth outcome and parenting. Once in the home, nurses were able to assess women for risks of eclamptic seizures and other pregnancy complications. When women at risk were identified, nurses made referrals for physician care to protect maternal and fetal outcome. Postpartum care provided support, maintained a clean environment, and followed mother and baby in an effort to identify risk, refer for early care, and educate mothers about infant feeding and child care (Fig. 1) [2].

Beginning in the 1850s, the relationship between proteinuria, edema, hyperreflexia, and impending eclamptic seizures was known. By 1900, hypertension had been added to the list, although it was not until the second decade of the twentieth century that nurses began to carry portable blood pressure cuffs into homes. Before that, nurses made sure that women at risk were seen in a clinic where stationary blood pressure equipment was available. The National Association of Public Health Nurses informed members through their journal about the work of prenatal services in member organizations [2]. In so doing, the journal helped to refine and spread this service, so that by 1916 prenatal and maternity care comprised between 18% to 24% of the visiting nurse caseload in two New York City agencies [3]. The Metropolitan Life Insurance Company felt that this care was so important to its members, that between 1916 and 1921 it reimbursed nursing agencies for these home visits. Between 1921 and 1929, the Shepard-Towner Maternity and Infancy Act funded almost 3000 visiting nurse prenatal and maternity services and over 3 million nurse home visits across the country [2–4].

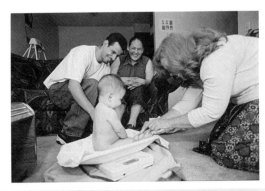

Fig. 1. Nurse with baby. (*From* the archives of the National Nurse Family Partnership; with permission.)

During prenatal home visits, nurses assessed for danger signs and educated women about headache, visual changes, edema, proteinuria, and epigastric pain. In their biweekly visits, nurses also educated women about diet, exercise, rest, preparation for delivery, infant feeding, and infant care (Fig. 2). As portable less expensive blood pressure cuffs became available, nurses began to take blood pressures at every visit.

Home-based prenatal care delivered by nurses had dual objectives. First, prenatal visitation was part of a national campaign to reduce high rates of maternal mortality. In 1900 in the United States, the rate of maternal mortality was 85 maternal deaths per 10,000 live births, and by 1930 it had only decreased to 67 maternal deaths per 10,000 live births. These rates were higher than those in

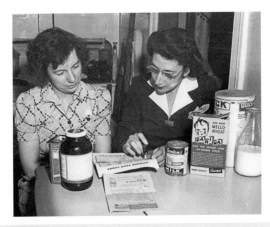

Fig. 2. Philadelphia Visiting Nurse doing newborn nutrition at home. (*From* the Barbara Bates Center for the Study of Nursing History, University of Pennsylvania School of Nursing; with permission.)

England and Wales, which had a rate of 48 maternal deaths per 10,000 live births in 1900 and 44 maternal deaths per 10,000 live births in 1930. Rates in Sweden and the Netherlands were even better, with a rate of 23 maternal deaths per 10,000 live births in 1900 and 34 maternal deaths per 10,000 live births in 1930 (Table 1) [5].

Second, the educational component of home visits was designed to Americanize the large numbers of immigrant women who arrived in the United States between 1900 and 1930 to American ways of homemaking and child care [6].

In 1920, Bertha Irons, RN, chief of field work at Boston School of Public Health Nursing, discussed prenatal nursing visits with immigrant women in the *Public Health Nurse*. Cognizant of the cultural and class differences between the nurse visitor and pregnant woman, Irons cautioned that the "[i]nitial visit is the most important one, for upon it depends the nurse's welcome for future visits and consequently her opportunity for helpfulness. . . .Having received the patient's permission for entering, let the visit proceed as a friendly call upon an acquaintance. . . . With a few guiding questions the patient will usually talk freely of her present pregnancy. . . . [7] This visit will afford an opportunity for observing the housing conditions and learning the economic situation of the family. . . . [The nurse] is a comfort to the lonely patient who has no other woman to talk to. . . ." [7] Mary Beard, RN [8,9], suggested that education on prenatal visits include discussions of rest and activity, exercise, diet, hygiene, hydration, preparation for childbirth, contents of the layette, signs and symptoms of labor, and what to expect at birth.

Nurses also provided written materials to supplement their teaching, frequently giving Mrs. Max West's booklet, Prenatal Care, published by the Federal Children's Bureau in 1913 [7]. Both Irons and Beard discussed the importance of assessing a women for complications of pregnancy by checking urine for protein, and the woman for edema, presence of headaches or visual changes. They also advised checking the condition of the mother's nipples, her gastrointestinal status, the nature of her vaginal discharge, and her work status. Over time, visiting nurses added assessment of blood pressure, fetal heart rate, and a woman's emotional status.

Physician-managed prenatal care, with assessment and education at regular intervals throughout pregnancy, did not become routine medical practice for

Table 1
Comparison of early twentieth century rates of maternal deaths

Country	Maternal deaths per 1000 live births 1900	Maternal deaths per 1000 live births 1930
United States	85	67
England and Wales	48	44
Sweden and the Netherlands	23	34

Data from: Loudon I. Death in childbirth: an international study of maternal mortality 1800–1950. Oxford (UK): Clarendon Press; 1992.

another 20 years, during which time nurses across the country were routinely providing, refining, and expanding their biweekly prenatal care. The first discussion of routine prenatal visits in an obstetric text occurred in 1923 and was a direct result of the experience of visiting nurses. At the urging of Mrs. Lowell Putnam, board chair of the Boston Instructive District Nursing Association, J. Whitridge Williams, MD, finally added a recommendation of routine prenatal office visits to his obstetrics text, Obstetrics. A Textbook for the Use of Students and Practitioners, 5th edition [10]. Thus, early twentieth century prenatal nurse-home visiting was a model and direct stimulus for physician-provided prenatal care. It can be argued that it was also a historical precursor of the NFP.

NURSE HOME VISITING 1978 TO PRESENT: THE NURSE FAMILY PARTNERSHIP
Randomized controlled trials

In 1977, Olds and colleagues implemented a randomized, controlled trial of a theory-driven nurse home visitation program for 400 pregnant women and new mothers in Elmira, New York [11,12]. Randomized, controlled trials also were conducted in Memphis, Tennessee, beginning in 1987 (N = 1135) [13,14], and Denver, beginning in 1994 (N = 735) [15,16]. Families in the Elmira trial were predominately white; those in the Memphis trial were predominately African American, and the Denver trial included families from diverse backgrounds including Mexican, white non-Mexican, European American, and African American. The Elmira and Memphis trials tested the efficacy of the nurse home visiting model. In Denver, the outcomes of women and children visited by either nurses or paraprofessionals using this model of visitation were compared.

All three trials enrolled women who were less than 26 weeks into their first pregnancy and had at least one of the following risk factors: younger than 19 years old, single, or low socioeconomic status. They were recruited from health department prenatal clinics, private obstetric offices, Planned Parenthood, public schools, and other community health and social service agencies. Visitation schedules evolved over the three trials, and by the last one in Denver, antepartum intervention began with weekly visits during the first month followed by biweekly home visits for the rest of pregnancy. Post partum, the nurse visited weekly during the first 6 weeks and then resumed by biweekly visits until 20 months. Between 20 and 24 months the nurse visited monthly. The following discussion looks only at outcomes in families visited by nurses, because families receiving the paraprofessional intervention had only one statistically significant outcome; mother child interaction was more responsive than in the control group [15].

The 15-year long-term follow-up for the Elmira participants demonstrated many long-lasting, significant, and positive outcomes of the intervention for the women and their children. Compared with the control groups, it was found that in families who received the 2.5-year visitation, there was:

- A decrease in contacts with the criminal justice system
- 69% fewer arrests among the women
- 81% reduction in convictions of the adolescent children
- 56% reduction in emergency room visits
- 32% reduction in subsequent pregnancies
- 83% increase in labor force participation among the mothers by the child's fourth birthday [11,17–19]

Further, a RAND corporation study showed a $4 return for every $1 invested in the intervention [20], and a cost–benefit analysis conducted at the request of the Washington state legislature projected a $17,180 lifetime cost savings for every child born to a mother who received 2.5 years of home visitation by a NFP nurse [21].

NATIONAL REPLICATION

As a result of excellent outcomes, the research team decided to replicate the intervention on a nationwide basis in a program now named the Nurse Family Partnership. As of May 2005, the program has been replicated in 20 states at 250 program sites that serve over 13,000 families a year. Program sites include local social service agencies; state, county, and city health departments; nurse-managed health centers; and visiting nurse associations. Each site creates teams that include one half-time supervisor for four full-time nurses who each carry a caseload of 25 families.

The intervention follows a standardized 2.5-year curriculum, and, like early twentieth century home-based prenatal nursing, the NFP is designed to improve pregnancy outcomes and child health and development. Additionally, Olds and colleagues realized that to achieve multi-generational changes in family health and social functioning, the program also would have to improve the skills and economic self-sufficiency of these vulnerable young women. Often pregnant by accident, they tend to have poor communication and life planning skills, and move in and out of relationships without forming lasting bonds. To achieve these goals, Olds grounded the NFP program in Bronfenbrenner's theory of human ecology, Bowlby's human attachment theory, and Bandura's theory of self-efficacy, because each provides insight into specific needs of this target population [22].

The theory of human ecology posits that child development is influenced by the characteristics and interactions of a family's social networks, neighborhood, and community. The theory of self-efficacy argues that individuals choose actions they are capable of and that they believe will achieve a desired result. Attachment theory is perhaps the best known and holds that, because of their biology, infants are predisposed to seek human closeness during times of stress. Success at forming a caring attachment with a primary caregiver results in a child's development of trust, empathy, and his or her own ability to parent later in life [22].

Based on these theories the NFP curriculum is designed to provide a therapeutic relationship between nurse and client in which a young mother learns effective decision-making, parenting, and problem-solving skills. She also learns to trust her expertise about herself and her children. In effect, the nurse mothers each young woman she works with, and in this role, the nurse models skills that the client incorporates into her own parenting and into her interactions with others in her environment, beginning with obstetric and pediatric providers. Most young mothers in this program have never had the kind of supportive relationship they have with their nurse. This program is client-focused. The importance of meeting a mother's goals is primary. It is the mother's agenda and not the nurse's that drives what happens in a home visit. In addition, the nurse works with a mother's personal support system to assist her as she completes her education and moves into the world of work. Building on a mother's strengths, the nurse helps each woman develop her sense of self-efficacy. Long after the program ends, the nurse's influence has a lasting impact on a family's health and welfare for generations to come.

During the course of the 2.5-year visitation, a nurse provides a mother with education across six domains: personal health; environmental health, maternal role, life course development, family and friends support networks, and health and human services. A young woman is educated about pregnancy, growth and development of the fetus and newborn, and ways to create a safe and stimulating environment for her young child. Together with the nurse, a client identifies her social supports and discusses strategies for strengthening and using this system to help her parent while progressing toward education and work goals. The mother is the expert on her own life. Nurses do not tell her what to do, but rather they respect and encourage her to make her own decisions and to use newly learned problem-solving strategies to achieve her heart's desires.

Using the model of behavioral change developed by Prochaska and colleagues [23], NFP nurses assess a client's stage of change, readiness to work on developing new behaviors, goal setting, and progress toward permanent change. Nurses understand that behavioral change must be an internal process to be successful. Therefore, they concentrate on supporting a client in her process of change rather than forcing change to take place. Most importantly, nurses try very hard to make sure that action steps for change are realistic and doable, so that self-efficacy is experienced and the change process is reinforced.

In the precontemplation stage of behavioral change, a woman is not interested in changing behavior, because, although she is aware of a problem, she may be unaware or unconcerned of the negative consequences for herself or her child or lacks motivation to change. She blames others and wishes others would change so her life will improve. When a nurse assesses that a woman is in the precontemplation stage, she focuses interventions to increase self-insight and move the client into the second phase, contemplation.

A woman may experience anxiety during the contemplation stage, because she has become aware that the problem is within and is ambivalent about taking the risk necessary for change. She tries to understand the causes and solutions but frequently falls into the yes but safety zone. As a nurse works with her client in this stage, she helps the woman look at the benefits of changing and the drawbacks of staying the same. When the woman decides the latter outweighs the former, she moves into the preparation phase and becomes committed to taking action, focusing less on the problem and more on an action plan.

The preparation phase is critical. Adequate time must be spent planning for change; otherwise the client is set up for failure and will return to old behaviors. She then must recycle through the beginning stages once again. In fact, lapses and failure, depending on the type of change being made, are discussed with the woman and normalized to avoid discouragement. With each attempt to change behavior, however, learning takes place, and change becomes an easier process.

During the action phase, the woman commits her time and energy to adapting new more effective behaviors. Over time there will be small steps backward, but after 3 to 6 months, new behaviors will become more common, and the woman will enter the maintenance phase. During this phase, lapses become fewer, and new behavior becomes routine and integrated into the woman's sense of self. A lifestyle alteration has occurred, and the woman is now in the sixth or final stage, self-empowerment. She has achieved her goal, adopted a new self-image, and achieved a new sense of self-efficacy. She now is living a healthier lifestyle and has no desire to return to the problem behavior pattern.

Fig. 3 diagrams a theoretical model of prenatal, birth, and program influences on future maternal behavior and child health and development that the NFP

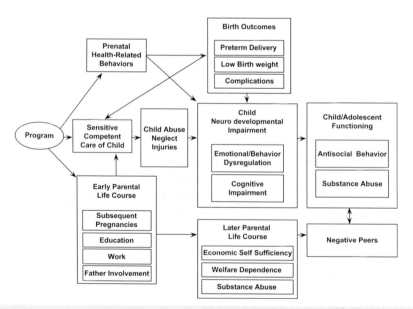

Fig. 3. Conceptual model of program influences on maternal and child development. (Reprinted from Olds D. Prenatal and infancy home visiting by nurses: from randomized trials to community replication. Prevention Science 2002;3(3):153–72; with permission.)

program is designed to influence. Nurses use interventions geared to facilitating prenatal and early parental and child life course behavioral change so that the potential for negative outcomes in pregnancy and child development is lessened. For instance, research has shown that prenatal exposure to tobacco, alcohol, and illegal drugs negatively affect the growth and development of the fetus, the potential for term birth, and increase the risk for neurobehavioral impairment of the child. Therefore, the program interventions place heavy emphasis on decreasing and eliminating use of these substances use during pregnancy.

Nurses in this home-based visitation program have a largely autonomous role providing education and case management for high-risk, low-income families living in complex environments. Therefore, fidelity to the model is important and is ensured as the program is replicated across the country in several ways. As nurses are hired into the program, they begin a standardized three-stage orientation and education program of more than 60 hours conducted by nurse educators from the national NFP. This curriculum is competency-based and prepares registered nurses to implement the NFP model of care.

The first stage has two steps, home study and group instruction. Just before attending a 3-day education session in Denver, nurses and supervisors complete a 20-hour self-study module. The home study module provides an introduction and foundation for understanding the theoretical basis of the program. In Denver, nurses and supervisors learn about the pregnancy intervention curriculum, and how to use the Visit-to-Visit program guidelines. They also learn about reflective practice, which incorporates supervision to help ensure fidelity to the program and to serve as a model for reflective communication and problem solving in work with clients.

Nurses have an hour of reflective supervision every week. The nurse brings client issues and concerns to the session for discussion so that she can return to a client with a fresh approach. The supervisor uses the sessions to assess how each nurse is doing and uses reflection to stimulate new ideas, approaches, and directions in the nurse's work. Reflective practice, which also includes case conferences and field supervision, provides a formal process of professional support and learning that enables nurses to develop the knowledge and competence necessary to deliver this complex model of care.

The second stage has two components, an NFP workshop and two Nursing Child Assessment (NCAST) training sessions. The 3-day NFP education workshop focuses on the infancy curriculum, how to use the Visit-to-Visit program guidelines, incorporating NCAST feeding and teaching assessments, Ages and Stages developmental assessments, and Partners in Parenting Education (PIPE) interventions. Either before or just after the second session, nurses and supervisors attend NCAST workshops and achieve proficiency in using NCAST feeding and teaching screening tools, which are used for assessing maternal child interaction from birth to 2 years.

PIPE is a curriculum designed to draw on the strengths of a parent to promote positive parenting skills and enhance the emotional connection between mother and baby. This program includes floor-time activities that help mothers learn to communicate with and teach their babies. Nurses begin to introduce these activities during home visits between birth and 2 years.

Floor time is an important part of each home visit during which a nurse asks the mother to put a blanket on the floor so they both can sit with the baby along with a doll that that each nurse brings to home visits. A nurse interacts with a doll so the baby does not give the nurse a reaction that he does not give to his mother. After creating relevance for a concept related to emotional connectedness or parenting, the nurse demonstrates communication or play with her doll and then asks the mother to try the activity with her baby.

In one lesson on mother/infant communication, the nurse first may hold her doll in her hands on its back so she is looking at the side of the doll's face. The nurse calls the doll's name and then slowly turns the doll's head to the sound of her voice. The nurse then smiles, turns her hands so the doll is facing her, and says something like, "Hello Sasha, did you hear me calling your name? Oh, I see you want to talk today. You are such a big boy. I see you need a rest. You have turned away (the nurse turns the doll's head slightly). I will wait until you are ready to talk some more." The nurse then asks the mother to hold her baby in the same way and call his name. The pleasure a new mother gets when her baby alerts to her voice and turns to see her is wonderful to see, and it stimulates further mother/child interaction. It also opens a discussion of what babies hear and see, the importance of infant stimulation, and the mother's central role as her baby's first teacher. Nurses use the NCAST assessment tools and Ages and Stages developmental assessment to plan targeted interventions with PIPE and other program materials designed to improve maternal child interactions, parenting skills, and child development.

The third stage also has two components: a workshop that focuses on the toddler curriculum and instruction on how to use the Visit-to-Visit guidelines, and the introduction of a unique curriculum Smart Choices. During the toddler period, nurses often focus on the mother's goals for the future as she prepares for termination at the baby's second birthday. Smart Choices was designed and integrated into the NFP curriculum to provide an additional approach to teaching problem-solving skills. These interactive lessons are based on student competencies developed in the academic field to prepare young adults to achieve life course goals for work or school success. The curriculum has 30 lessons, which are in the narrative form of a story and discussion designed to build communication, thinking, organizational, technology, and workforce skills. It is also designed to strengthen the ability to use community resources and build personal support networks. Nurses are encouraged to use Smart Choices with clients who need to work on these specific skills.

Nationally, the NFP collects data from replication sites through a Web-based Clinical Information System that monitors the work and client outcomes of each program. Nurses collect data that are entered on each home visit and on maternal smoking patterns, pregnancy outcomes, timing of subsequent pregnancies, the child's growth and development, childhood injuries, reported child abuse and neglect, and the mother's status in terms of education, work, and use of welfare. These data are analyzed and returned to local NFP sites to provide them with evidence of their progress toward program goals and outcome, and to inform individual nurse practice trends and for quality improvement measures. In this way, outcomes at each site are measured against national benchmarks, and sites use this information to improve the service they provide. Data also are used with national and state legislators to lobby for funding, and with other funding sources to obtain required match. Several states, including Pennsylvania, Colorado, Louisiana, and Oklahoma, have committed to a statewide initiative, developing and funding sites statewide.

Continuing education and clinical consultation are on-going parts of the program and are designed by nurse clinical consultants from the national NFP office or employed by a state initiative. This can take the form of regular conference calls with supervisors, with teams at several sites, and state or regional conferences with guest speakers and workshops. Nurses are also responsible for their own growth as home visitors. The NFP has developed a competency-based assessment program. Through the supervisory process, nurses set annual competency-based goals, steps for monitoring goal attainment, and with the supervisor, engage in periodic assessment of their progress.

SUMMARY

Nurse home visiting with pregnant women and new mothers in the early decades of the twentieth century was designed to improve birth and newborn outcomes, hasten Americanization of immigrant mothers, and improve their parenting skills (Fig. 4). Today the NFP home visitation program improves newborn and child outcomes by positively influencing maternal role attainment and significantly decreasing maternal smoking and other substance abuse, child abuse and neglect, and children's emergency room visits. It also improves life possibilities for vulnerable young women by decreasing the interval and frequency of subsequent pregnancies and reduces dependence on welfare by increasing workforce participation. The program's effects do not end with the intervention. Long term follow-up in randomized controlled clinical trials has shown that in adolescence children whose mothers were participants in the NFP intervention had fewer arrests and convictions, less drug use, and fewer sexual partners.

Nurse-home visiting has always been a practice with a higher level of independent nursing assessment and decision-making. Over time, this nursing practice has been implemented by independent nursing organizations such VNAs, nurse-run settlement houses, and nurse-managed centers. Today the NFP outcomes show that this program of home visitation, which is grounded in theories of child development, attachment, and behavioral change, has the potential for reducing the damaging and widespread problems experienced by low-income, vulnerable women and their children. As a result, four states have committed to initiatives funding statewide replication of this program, and together with 19 other states without statewide initiatives, have developed replication sites in 250 counties nationwide. Today, Olds and colleagues in national and regional

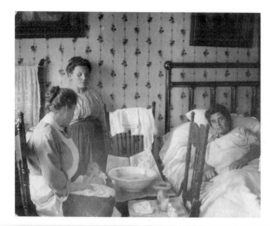

Fig. 4. Philadelphia Visiting Nurse at a postpartum visit. (*From* the Barbara Bates Center for the Study of Nursing History, University of Pennsylvania School of Nursing; with permission.)

offices, and NFP nurse home visitors around the country, work toward the goal of making this program available to every vulnerable family in the United States. Nurses, by maintaining fidelity to the NFP model, ensure that its impact continues to change the life course trajectory for multiple generations of families.

Acknowledgements

The authors want to acknowledge and thank the staff members at the Prevention Research Center, the National Nurse Family Partnership, Denver, and the Barbara Bates Center for the Study of the History of Nursing for their contributions to this article.

References

[1] Enkiji MS. Innovative program offers guidance, hope: the Nurse Family Partnership pairs nurses with mothers-to-be. It has been described as one of the state's "best kept secrets." Sacramento Bee May 13, 2005. p. 1.
[2] Dawley K. Ideology and self-interest: nursing, medicine, and the elimination of the midwife. Nurs Hist Rev 2001;9:99–126.
[3] Halsey OS. Health insurance and public health nursing. Public Health Nurse Quarterly 1916;8(3):58–66.
[4] Frankel L, Dublin L. Visiting nurse and life insurance: a statistical summary of results for eight years. Reprinted in the Quarterly Publications of the American Statistical Association. June 1918.
[5] Loudon I. Death in childbirth: an international study of maternal care and maternal mortality 1800–1950. Oxford (England): Clarendon Press; 1992.
[6] Buhler-Wilkerson K. No place like home: a history of nursing and home care in the United States. Baltimore (MD): The Johns Hopkins University Press; 2001.
[7] Irons B. Prenatal nursing. Public Health Nurs 1920;12(6):594–601.
[8] Beard M. Prenatal Nursing. Public Health Nurse Quarterly 1923;15(8):415.
[9] Beard M. Prenatal nursing. Public Health Nurse Quarterly 1915;7:313–24.

[10] Longo LD, Thomsen CM. Prenatal care and its evolution in America. Presented at the Second Motherhood Symposium of the Women's Studies Research Center, University of Wisconsin. Madison, Wisconsin, April 9–10, 1981.

[11] Olds DL, Henderson CR, Cole R, et al. Long-term effects of nurse home visitation on children's criminal and antisocial behavior: 15-year follow-up of a randomized controlled trial. JAMA 1998;280(14):1238–44.

[12] Eckenrode J, Ganzel B, Henderson CR, et al. Preventing child abuse and neglect with a program of nurse home visitation: the limiting effects of domestic violence. JAMA 2000; 282(11):1385–91.

[13] Kitzman H, Olds DL, Sidora K, et al. Enduring effects of nurse home visitation on maternal course: a 3-year follow-up of a randomized trial. JAMA 2000;28(315):1983–9.

[14] Olds DL, Kitzman H, Cole R, et al. Effects of nurse home visiting on maternal life course and child development: age 6 follow-up results of a randomized trial. Pediatrics 2004;114(6): 1550–9.

[15] Olds DL, Robinson J, O'Brian R, et al. Home visiting by paraprofessionals and by nurses: a randomized, controlled trial. Pediatrics 2002;110(3):486–96.

[16] Olds DL, Robinson J, Pettitt LM, et al. Effects of home visits by paraprofessionals and by nurses: age 4 follow-up results of a randomized trial. Pediatrics 2004;114(6):1560–8.

[17] Yeager C. Testimony before House Committee on Appropriations Subcommittee on Departments of Labor Health & Human Services, Education and Related Agencies April 14, 2005.

[18] National Nurse Family Partnership. Fact Sheet. Available at: http://www.nursefamilypartnership.org homepage and research evidence. Accessed October 10, 2005.

[19] Olds DL, Henderson CR Jr, Chamberlin R, et al. Preventing child abuse and neglect: fifteen-year follow-up of a randomized trial. JAMA 1997;278(8):637–43.

[20] Karoly LA, Greenwood PW, Everingham SS, et al. Investing in our children: what we know and don't know about the costs and benefits of early childhood interventions. Santa Monica (CA): The RAND Corporation; 1998.

[21] Aos S, Lieb R, Mayfield J, et al. Benefits and costs of prevention and early intervention programs for youth, Olympia (WA): Washington State Institute for Public Policy; 2004.

[22] Olds D. Prenatal and infancy home visiting by nurses: from randomized trials to community replication. Prev Sci 2002;3(3):153–72.

[23] Prochaska JO, Norcross JC, DiClemente CC. Changing for good. New York: Avon Books; 1994.

Nurs Clin N Am 40 (2005) 817–829

NURSING CLINICS
OF NORTH AMERICA

Using the Omaha System to Document the Wellness Needs of the Elderly

Lisa Ann Plowfield, RN, PhD*,
Evelyn R. Hayes, PhD, APRN, BC,
Bethany Hall-Long, PhD, RNC, FAAN

School of Nursing, College of Health Sciences,
University of Delaware, 250 North College Avenue, Newark, DE 19716, USA

H ealth promotion for the elderly occurs in many sites, and the activities vary based on the provider of service and the site. Health fairs frequently provide blood pressure screening, glucose and cholesterol testing, stroke risk assessments, depression and anxiety screenings, and specific cancer screening and education. Older adults many times access multiple sites of free services to monitor their health and receive information on various health topics. As access to services often is limited for the elderly, health promotion and education activities within the community can be an important resource for monitoring and early intervention with referrals to appropriate providers.

With a grant from the US Public Health Service Division of Nursing, the University of Delaware (UD) Nursing Center developed an ongoing community resource for health promotion, education, and disease screening activities for vulnerable populations (1D1HP00239-01). The targeted populations were the homeless and elderly in this 2-year grant project. Based on previous experience and the history of data management at the UD Nursing Center, the staff recognized very early in the project the need to document one-time, site-of-care outcome data. Using the Omaha System (OS) of documentation, the staff created paper surveys that student nurses and center staff used to collect data in a standardized format for future analysis. This article presents an academic center's use of the OS and the challenges of documenting the outcomes of one-time contacts with clients during health promotion, education, and disease screening events.

This work was supported by: US PHS Division of Nursing #1D1HP00239-01 Corresponding author for proof and reprints:

*Corresponding author. E-mail address: plow@udel.edu (L.A. Plowfield).

UNIVERSITY OF DELAWARE NURSING CENTER

Established in 1995 with a 5-year Health Resources and Services Administration grant (1D10NU30224-01), the UD Nursing Center is a nurse-managed center that serves vulnerable populations, especially the community dwelling elderly throughout the state. The UD Nursing Center provides comprehensive geriatric assessments for families with frail elders and health promotion, education, and disease screening services. These services usually are provided at sites where the elderly, homeless, and urban living can access them easily; some sites include senior high-rise apartment buildings, community centers, homeless shelters, and senior centers. The center is staffed by two faculty and students. Most outreach health contacts are provided by students during their clinical coursework. The center remains a grant-funded initiative with staffing support from the UD Department of Nursing. Multiple sources, private, state, and federal, have financed the outreach health services and related research and program evaluation activities.

REVIEW OF LITERATURE

Health services for vulnerable populations

Health promotion and disease prevention programs are essential health services to reduce health care costs and improve quality of life for vulnerable populations [1,2]. Although the risk of disease increases with age or homelessness, poor health does not have to be a result of either demographic. A healthy lifestyle is more influential than genetic factors in preventing the deterioration of older adults' health [3]. Populations with a lack of resources such as the homeless and elderly have made it difficult to implement and measure health promotion outcomes, but these are highly recommended [4].

Nurse-run centers and academic–community outreach have been found to decrease costs and improve the vulnerable populations' reports of health. Badger and McArthur [5] studied the impact of health promotion and disease screening efforts at a nurse- and student nurse-run clinic in a low-income public housing complex, whose residents were mostly elderly minority women. Over 693 vulnerable visits were made, focusing on blood pressure monitoring, health education, mental health screenings and referrals, pain management, and diabetes management. Health outcomes improved dramatically, with costs savings of $36,000 in the first year from the program's operation.

Nunez and colleagues [6] operated a community-based senior health promotion program using a collaborative practice model. The partnership is a nurse-managed wellness center that provides service for suburban, low-income, minority populations. Their interventions were based upon Healthy People 2010 [7] and were designed specifically for frail elders. Interventions included blood pressure screenings, group fitness classes, first aid, safety, self-care management, and nutrition. Their health promotion measures resulted in reports of improved physical and mental health status, performance roles, and social functioning as compared with national norms. Doctor visits and hospitalizations were reported almost half as frequently among those who received these services.

Nationally, one in seven Americans is diagnosed with chronic physical or mental illness, representing 78% of total health care spending [8]. Elderly people who are physically active, eat healthy, and avoid tobacco, have half the rate of disability of those who do not take these measures [9]. Chronic illness prevention is an essential component of health promotion, and effective strategies often are underused [8].

Issues in capturing data

Data collection with vulnerable populations in the community setting presents unique opportunities and challenges [10]. Client interactions with health education and promotion program measures are often episodic and short-term in nature. Many are conducted as one-time screenings or health fairs. Thus, these episodes of care present challenges for tool development or application and data collection [10].

When working with vulnerable populations, it is imperative that surveys be concise, direct, and provide opportunity for expanded responses [11,12]. Nursing students and faculty, working in episodic, community-based care settings need to be educated as to the use of specific tools to enhance reliability of the tools' usages, and to ensure that patients receive the most appropriate education and timely referrals [10].

The literature reflects a surge in community–academic partnerships that offer creative health promotion programs while providing beneficial services to clients and students [13]. These programs need to address real community problems and have data collection tools and systems in place that are culturally sensitive, capture benefit and cost outcomes, provide a base for service–research learning, and integrate training on how to apply the tools in the field [14,15].

Omaha System of documentation

The UD Nursing Center staff selected the OS for documenting the outcomes of care. This documentation system is research-based with interdisciplinary language, making it applicable to all health care providers. The system maintains a standardized language and is one of 13 recognized systems for documentation of health data by the American Nurses Association [16]. The OS offers a full range of applications including client, family, community, populations, and acute, chronic, and primary care. The OS allows for data recording from assessment through all phases of care. In addition, this system is adaptable to pencil and paper and computerized systems.

The structure of the OS includes the four domains of needs (or problems), problem classification, problem rating scale, outcome ratings, and an intervention schema. A brief description of each component follows. The domains of needs are: environmental, physiological, psychosocial, and health related behaviors. Problem classification follows based on symptoms and risk factors. Problems can be classified as a:

- Deficit or impairment (indicates client has signs or symptoms requiring attention)

- Potential deficit (risk factors exist that may lead to an actual impairment)
- Adequate (no symptoms or risk factors evident)
- Health promotion (client desires a change or an improvement with the need) [16]

Each problem has a standardized list of signs and symptoms for ease of data recording. This standardized list allows providers to collect and view cohort data easily and with enhanced accuracy.

After all problems are identified and signs and symptoms documented, the provider uses the Problem Rating Scale to document the client's current knowledge, behavior, and status related to the identified need. Knowledge is the client's ability to remember and interpret information. Behavior is the client's observable responses, actions, or activities fitting the occasion or purpose. Status is the client's condition in relation to objective and subjective defining characteristics [16]. The rating scale is used only on those problems in which a client has evidenced a need or when a potential need that requires intervention exists. The outcome ratings are indicated on a five-point Likert scale, with one low and five high.

A standardized format and list within the OS are used to document interventions. Four categories of interventions are noted with a standardized list of targets. The categories are surveillance (usual monitoring of the client's status [eg, blood pressure monitoring]); health teaching, guidance, or counseling (eg, family planning); case management; or technical procedures (eg, use of nebulizer, dressing change) [16].

SURVEY DEVELOPMENT

While appreciating the comprehensiveness of the OS, the project team saw a need to have a short focused survey for use at various community events including health fairs. This need heralded the development of three focused surveys. Based on the needs of the population served, three short surveys were designed for the health promotion and disease screening outreach services. The selected areas for survey development were blood pressure/stroke risk screening, nutrition, and general health inventory.

The project team designed the initial versions of the three surveys. Several considerations guided content development and layout design. The major considerations for content were demographics (using the standardized and accepted demographic data categories of the National Nursing Centers Consortium) and use of selected needs of the OS. For the blood pressure and stroke risk screening survey, the OS needs that had the highest relevance and impact were circulation, respiration, prescription medication regimen, and communication with community resources. For the nutrition screening survey, the team incorporated the American Dietetics Association Nutrition Screening Tool, a diet history, and the OS needs of nutrition and communication with community resources. The third tool developed was a general health inventory survey. This tool incorporated the SF-12 Health Status Questionnaire and the OS needs of social contact, physical activity, and emotional stability. Content relevance was based on previous health screening activities that had been provided to the homeless and elderly in earlier initiatives.

In addition to the specific content, each of the screening surveys included all the elements of the four domains (physiological, psychological, environmental, and health-related) and the primary rating scale for outcomes (knowledge, behavior, status). Nurse experts with OS and health screening expertise reviewed the selected components for the surveys. The project team and expert reviewers worked until they had 100% agreement.

Once the initial content was identified, survey layout was pursued by the team. A simple-to-use, paper-and-pencil tool that allowed for easy duplication was developed. Using a standard 8.5 × 11 in paper size, each survey was developed using one page folded in half to create a four-sided booklet of 5.5 × 8.5 in. The demographics were noted on the front page, the major content areas on the two center pages, and the OS-specific information for referencing on the fourth and final page of the booklet. Figs. 1 to 4 show each page layout of the Blood Pressure/Stroke Risk Screening Survey.

IMPLEMENTATION

All students previously had been introduced and educated on the OS in the junior year, and a group of 12 senior students routinely used this system of documentation during their final preceptored community-based clinical experience. Students were supervised in the use of the tools by faculty. The students were to submit the completed tools weekly, and they were reviewed and examined at the end of the semester. In using the survey tool during this pilot period, 57 blood pressure/stroke risk screening, 17 nutrition, and 68 general health inventory surveys were completed and submitted. The data then were entered into spreadsheets for analysis of the community needs in these targeted areas. In addition, the completion of the tools and the information gathering was reviewed by the project team.

The most common area of complete information was the demographic data. The second area in which documentation was complete was the second page of all surveys. This page had the most essential information related to the purpose for the survey and outreach health activity. The third and four pages of the survey were related areas, in which areas of need might be found. These pages frequently were not completed or had multiple areas of missing data.

In examining the pilot data of the 57 blood pressure/stroke risk screening surveys, five clients were identified as having impairment in this area. As required by the OS format, the problem rating scale was completed. In two cases in which impairment did not exist, a student nurse completed the outcome ratings, indicating that he or she did not understand the documentation format completely. In addition, in three cases, a finding of edema existed, indicating an area of impairment, and the impairment was not documented as such. One area of the survey, Communication with Community Resources, had unusable data. In a few cases, this section was not completed; many clients who

Promoting Healthy Lifestyles in Delaware Project

BP/Stroke Risk Screening

DEMOGRAPHICS (circle all that apply)

Year of birth: _____   **Date:** _____   **Gender: M — F**

Race:
1—White   2—Black   3—American Indian/Eskimo/Aleut
4—Asian/Pacific Islander   5—other   6—unknown

Ethnicity:
1—Hispanic origin   2—Non-Hispanic origin   3—unknown

Marital Status:
1—single   2—married   3—separated
4—divorced   5—domestic partner   6—widowed
7—common law partner   8—other   9—unknown

Primary Language Spoken:
1—English   2—Spanish   3—other

Employment Status:
1—full-time   2—part-time
3—unemployed/seeking work   4—unemployed not seeking work
5—retired   6—student
7—disabled   8—other
9—unknown

Household Size: _____   (enter numeric value)

Highest Grade Completed:
1—no education   2—less than 8th grade
3—some high school   4—GED high school equivalency diploma
5—high school graduate   6—some technical or trade school
8—some college   7—technical or trade school graduate
9—college graduate   10—any post-graduate work
11—unknown

Citizenship Status:
1—US citizen   2—not a US citizen   3—Unknown

Usual Source of Health Care:
1—nursing center   2—other physician/nurse
3—city district health center 4—community health center
5—emergency room   6—none
7—unknown

Fig. 1. Front page of survey.

Heart Rate: _____   **Rhythm:** (circle one) Regular / Irregular

BP: _____   (circle one) sitting / standing / lying)

Edema: _____

Other Data/Risk Factors: _____

_____

CIRCULATION

Modifiers: (select one)
Adequate   Health Promotion   Potential   Impairment

Signs/Symptoms of Impairment: (select those that apply)
1—edema   2—cramping
3—decreased pulses   4—discoloration of skin/cyanosis
5—temperature change in affected area   6—varicosities
7—syncopal episodes   8—abnormal BP
9—pulse deficit   10—irregular heart rate
11—excessively rapid heart rate   12—excessively slow heart rate
13—anginal pain   14—abnormal heart sounds/
15—other   murmurs

Problem Rating Scale for Outcomes: (rate from 1 to 5)
Knowledge _____   **Behavior** _____   **Status** _____

PRESCRIBED MEDICATION REGIMEN

Modifiers: (select one)
Adequate   Not Applicable   Health Promotion   Potential

Meds Reviewed : Yes ☐   No ☐   Meds in Home: Yes ☐   No ☐
Plan to Obtain/Refill_____
Lacks Knowledge of Med:
  ☐ actions   ☐ dose   ☐ side effects   ☐ adm./adm.by:_____

Signs/Symptoms of Impairment: (select those that apply)
1—deviates from prescribed dosage/   4—improper storage of medication
   schedule   5—unable/unwilling to perform
2—demonstrates side-effects   procedure
3—inadequate system for taking   6—fails to obtain immunization
   medication   7—other

Problem Rating Scale for Outcomes: (rate from 1 to 5)
Knowledge _____   **Behavior** _____   **Status** _____

Fig. 2. Second page of survey.

RESPIRATION

Modifiers: (select one)
Adequate   Health Promotion   Potential   Impairment

Rate: _____   **Pattern:** _____

Lung sounds: _____

Other Data/Risk Factors: _____

_____

Signs/Symptoms of Impairment: (circle all that apply)

1—abnormal breath patterns   2—unable to breathe independently
3—cough   4—unable to cough/expectorate
5—cyanosis   independently
6—abnormal sputum   7—noisy respirations
8—rhinorrhea   9—abnormal breath sounds
10—other

Problem Rating Scale for Outcomes: (rate from 1 to 5)
Knowledge _____   Behavior _____   Status _____

COMMUNICATION WITH COMMUNITY RESOURCES

Modifiers: (select one)
Adequate   Health Promotion   Potential   Impairment

Food Resources: _____

Transportation Resources: _____

Other Data/Risk Factors: _____

_____

Signs/Symptoms of Impairment: (circle all that apply)
1—unfamiliar with options/procedures   2—difficulty understanding roles/
   or obtaining services   regulations of service providers
3—unable to communicate concerns   4—dissatisfaction with services
   to service providers   5—language barrier
6—inadequate/unavailable resources   7—other

Problem Rating Scale for Outcomes: (rate from 1 to 5)
Knowledge _____   Behavior _____   Status _____

Fig. 3. Third page of survey.

Problem Classification Scheme (Circle all that apply)

Domain I: Environmental
1. Income
2. Sanitation
3. Residence
4. Neighborhood/workplace safety
5. Other

Domain II: Psychosocial
6. Communication with community resources
7. Social contact
8. Role change
9. Interpersonal relationship
10. Spiritual distress
11. Grief
12. Emotional stability
13. Human sexuality
14. Care taking/parenting
15. Neglected child/adult
16. Abused child/adult
17. Growth and development
18. Other

Sources: **SF-12 Health Status Questionnaire
+The Omaha System, 1992

Domain III: Physiological
19. Hearing
20. Vision
21. Speech and language
22. Dentition
23. Cognition
24. Pain
25. Consciousness
26. Integument
27. Neuro-musculo-skeletal function
28. Respiration
29. Circulation
30. Digestion-hydration
31. Bowel function
32. Genito-urinary function
33. Antepartum/postpartum
34. Other

Domain IV: Health Related Behaviors
35. Nutrition
36. Sleep and rest patterns
37. Physical activity
38. Personal hygiene
39. Substance misuse
40. Family planning
41. Health care supervision
42. Prescribed medication regimen
43. Technical procedure
44. Other

Problem Rating Scale for Outcomes:
Knowledge: The ability of the client to remember and interpret information

1	2	3	4	5
No knowledge	Minimal knowledge	Basic knowledge	Adequate knowledge	Superior knowledge

Behavior: The observable responses, actions, or activities of the client fitting the occasion or purpose

1	2	3	4	5
Not appropriate	Rarely appropriate	Inconsistently appropriate	Usually appropriate	Consistently appropriate

Status: The condition of the client in relation to objective and subjective defining characteristics

1	2	3	4	5
Extreme Signs/Symptoms	Severe Signs/Symptoms	Moderate Signs/Symptoms	Minimal Signs/Symptoms	No Signs/Symptoms

Fig. 4. Back page of survey.

had evidence of need were coded incorrectly as having no impairment. The importance of cohort data from episodic visits is described in the pilot case analysis of 57 clients who completed the blood pressure/stroke risk screening survey (Box 1).

DISCUSSION

Documentation of care needs in community dwelling vulnerable populations was conducted during various scheduled UD Nursing Center outreach activities. Using the OS as a basis for need targeted surveys, faculty and students had an effective and efficient paper-based documentation system. The use of the

---

Box 1: Case study analysis

Blood pressure and stroke risk assessment of vulnerable populations: a University of Delaware Nursing Center pilot study

Fifty-seven community dwelling homeless and elderly clients participated in the University of Delaware's nursing student health outreach assessment. Twenty-three men and 34 women participated. The mean age was 73.12 years (SD 11.68), with a range of 41 to 92 years. The sample was mostly white (63%), followed by black. One third of the clients were married; 28% were widowed; 21% were single, and 5% each had separated or divorced.

English was the primary language spoken by 95% of clients. Fifty-eight percent were retired. Eight were unemployed, with six seeking work. The mean household size was 1.7 (SD 1.07), with a range of one to five. Thirty-three percent reported living alone. The clients, in general, were well-educated, with 40% having a high school diploma, and 31% with education beyond high school. Most (79%) received their health care from a primary care provider, and 5.2% indicated they had no source of primary health care. Other sources of care were community health centers, city health centers and the emergency room.

When examining the heart rate and blood pressure of these 57 clients, the mean heart rate was 71.18 (SD 9.3), with a range of 54 to 100 beats per minute. Blood pressure had a mean of 129.5 mm Hg systolic (SD 15.69) and 74.21 mm Hg diastolic (SD 9.52). The systolic range was 100 to 170, and the diastolic range was 50 to 110. Using the JNC VII guidelines for classifying blood pressure, the systolic readings indicated 22.8% were within normal hypertension, stage 2 (Fig. 5).

Using the OS of documentation, five clients had impairment in circulation documented. The predominant sign was that of edema. In examining their circulation needs as shown by the participants' knowledge, behavior, and status ratings, the knowledge scores ranged from one to three on a scale of five (with five being the highest level of knowledge). Most clients with ratings had a behavior rating of three to four. Status of this need ranged from two to three. The sample size is too small to analyze beyond descriptive analysis. With these 57 patients, no prescribed medication regimen impairments were noted. Respiration had one impairment documented and was noted by decreased breath sounds and cough. Several clients had reported an interest in improving their health and knowledge about their medications, resulting in a need classification of health promotion using the OS.

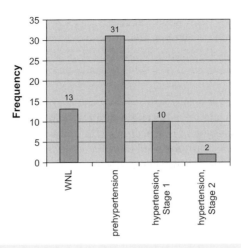

Fig. 5. Hypertension levels of blood pressure screening participants.

surveys to document needs of elderly clients in the community had multiple strengths. The survey format guided nursing students with their assessment of clients. The information collected was focused, and the tool allowed for identifying additional client needs, which enhanced student skill development and organization with health screenings. The survey was easy to read and complete. The format promoted documentation of relevant client information in a timely manner. Meaningful interactions between nursing students and the clients were enhanced by the OS-related surveys while providing practical screening activities that were not overly time consuming. Use of the surveys incorporating relevant portions of the OS provided focus for the student assessment and documentation of client needs.

Applicable to use in various community settings, the surveys allowed for analysis of the cohort perspective of needs in the targeted areas with elders who attend community events including health fairs. The surveys captured participant demographic information so that the populations served could be identified. Assessment results and care provided were recorded easily. In this pilot implementation, the targeted conditions for the nursing outreach activities were chronic illnesses, with a focus on cardiovascular disease, cancer, and diabetes mellitus. The comprehensive OS allows providers to select targeted needs for efficient documentation. Other known health needs, especially chronic conditions such as depression, are suitable for assessment and documentation using the OS.

The primary limitation of this pilot implementation was the need for greater in-service and education about the use of the surveys to ensure consistency of data collection. Doutrich and Hall-Long [14,15] also noted the critical importance of education and training users of the tools in the practice setting. In the pilot study, the section with most data recording errors was

Communication with Community Resources. In addition to an incomplete understanding of the OS of documentation, this area may have been more difficult to interpret by the student nurses. This type of information required a higher level of analysis. The clients were community dwelling elders and homeless; therefore, information was more difficult and challenging to collect. In addition, although it was not the intent of this endeavor, the data collection did not allow for follow-up with clients. Clients, however, were provided with educational information and follow-up referral contacts for those who did not have a current health care provider.

Data management is crucial to the successful outcome of any project. This pilot experience with data collection was challenging and provided lessons learned. The user-friendly surveys had multiple data points to be collected. Missing data, unusable data, and incomplete data presented distractions from getting the most targeted and comprehensive assessment of the client's health needs. These inconsistencies in data collection demonstrate the need for orientation, monitoring, and addressing on-going learning needs related to the OS.

Martin [16] reported that client data too often end up buried in the data cemetery. Of course, this is not a desired outcome and may happen because data management requires special skills and planning from inception of the project. The meaningful data collected with the OS can be used to address client's needs and services to meet those needs reliably. Data collected from the 57 clients using the blood pressure/stroke risk survey demonstrated the need for continued screening, health promotion education, follow-up monitoring for those with varying levels of hypertension, and referrals for treatment.

This pilot program and use of targeted record keeping using the OS demonstrated the power of information for both students and faculty. This project served educational nursing needs also. Faculty expressed that conferences with the students after data collection proved to be an ideal time to evaluate the goals for the screening and education activities. The findings of this pilot study are reflective of the findings of Mauer and Smith [10]. Based on these assessments, the faculty and students discussed the need for and design of future and follow-up outreach activities.

Information, the key source of evidence-based care, needs to be incorporated into all nursing care. Outreach health services and community care projects can be analyzed, and the need for this type of care within the local community can be understood more fully. Therefore, the OS can be used to provide efficient and targeted health survey data on populations.

Acknowledgments

The authors thank additional project staff involved in this work: Michelle Provost-Craig, PhD; Marianne Carter, MS, RD; Jean E. Raymond, RN, MSN; Joyce Witte, and Kathleen Williamson, RN, MSN.

References
[1] Centers for Disease Control and Prevention. Healthy aging: preventing disease and improving quality of life among older Americans. Atlanta (GA): Centers for Disease Control and Prevention; 2001.
[2] Resnick B. Health promotion practices of older adults: model testing. Public Health Nursing 2003;20(1):2–12.
[3] Minkler M, Schauffler H, Clements-Nolle K. Health promotion for older Americans in the 21st century. Am J Health Promot 2000;14(6):371–9.
[4] Power R, French R, Connelly J, et al. Health, health promotion, and homeless. BMJ 1999;318(2):590–2.
[5] Badger T, McArthur D. Academic nursing clinic: impact on health and costs outcomes for vulnerable populations. Appl Nurs Res 2003;16(1):60–4.
[6] Nunez D, Armbuster C, Phillips W, et al. Community based senior health promotion program using a collaborative practice model, the Escalante health partnerships. Public Health Nursing 2003;20(20):25–32.
[7] United States Department of Health and Human Services. Healthy People 2010. Washington (DC): United States Department of Health and Human Services; 2000.
[8] Council of State Governments. State officials' guide to chronic illness. Lexington (KY): Council of State Governments; 2003. Available at: http://www.csg.org/CSG/Policy/health/chronic+illness/state+officials+guide+to+chronic+illness.htm.
[9] Resnick B. Health promotion practices of the old-old. J Am Acad Nurse Pract 1998;10(4):147–53.
[10] Maurer FA, Smith CM. Community/public health nursing practice. 3rd edition. Philadelphia: WB Saunders; 2005.
[11] Smith J. Education and public health. Alexandria (VA): Association for Curriculum Development; 2003.
[12] Wurzbach M. Communitypublic health education and promotion: a guide to program design and evaluation. Gaithersburg (MD): Aspen; 2002.
[13] Lancaster J. From the editor. Education and practice: partners in improving public health. Fam Community Health 2004;27(4):280.
[14] Doutrich D. Education and practice: Dynamic partners for improving cultural competence in public health. Fam Community Health 2004;27(4):298–307.
[15] Hall-Long B. Partners in action: a public health program for baccalaureate nursing students. Fam Community Health 2004;27(4):338–45.
[16] Martin K. The Omaha System, A key to practice, documentation, and information management. 2nd edition. St. Louis (MO): Elsevier; 2005.

Nurs Clin N Am 40 (2005) 831–854

NURSING CLINICS
OF NORTH AMERICA

ELSEVIER
SAUNDERS

CUMULATIVE INDEX 2005

Note: Page numbers of article titles are in **boldface** type.

United States Postal Service
Statement of Ownership, Management, and Circulation

1. Publication Title	2. Publication Number	3. Filing Date
Nursing Clinics of North America	0 0 2 9 - 6 4 6 5	9/15/05

4. Issue Frequency	5. Number of Issues Published Annually	6. Annual Subscription Price
Mar, Jun, Sep, Dec	4	$100.00

7. Complete Mailing Address of Known Office of Publication (Not printer) (Street, city, county, state, and ZIP+4)

Elsevier Inc.
6277 Sea Harbor Drive
Orlando, FL 32887-4800

Contact Person
Gwen C. Campbell

Telephone
215-239-3685

8. Complete Mailing Address of Headquarters or General Business Office of Publisher (Not printer)

Elsevier Inc., 360 Park Avenue South, New York, NY 10010-1710

9. Full Names and Complete Mailing Addresses of Publisher, Editor, and Managing Editor (Do not leave blank)

Publisher (Name and complete mailing address)

Tim Griswold, Elsevier Inc., 1600 John F. Kennedy Blvd., Suite 1800, Philadelphia, PA 19103-2899

Editor (Name and complete mailing address)

Maria Lorusso, Elsevier Inc., 1600 John F. Kennedy Blvd., Suite 1800, Philadelphia, PA 19103-2899

Managing Editor (Name and complete mailing address)

Heather Cullen, Elsevier Inc., 1600 John F. Kennedy Blvd., Suite 1800, Philadelphia, PA 19103-2899

10. Owner (Do not leave blank. If the publication is owned by a corporation, give the name and address of the corporation immediately followed by the names and addresses of all stockholders owning or holding 1 percent or more of the total amount of stock. If not owned by a corporation, give the names and addresses of the individual owners. If owned by a partnership or other unincorporated firm, give its name and address as well as those of each individual owner. If the publication is published by a nonprofit organization, give its name and address.)

Full Name	Complete Mailing Address
Wholly owned subsidiary of	4520 East-West Highway
Reed/Elsevier Inc., US holdings	Bethesda, MD 20814

11. Known Bondholders, Mortgagees, and Other Security Holders Owning or Holding 1 Percent or More of Total Amount of Bonds, Mortgages, or Other Securities. If none, check box ☐ None

Full Name	Complete Mailing Address
N/A	

12. Tax Status (For completion by nonprofit organizations authorized to mail at nonprofit rates) (Check one)
The purpose, function, and nonprofit status of this organization and the exempt status for federal income tax purposes:
☐ Has Not Changed During Preceding 12 Months
☐ Has Changed During Preceding 12 Months (Publisher must submit explanation of change with this statement)

(See Instructions on Reverse)

PS Form 3526, October 1999

13. Publication Title	14. Issue Date for Circulation Data Below
Nursing Clinics of North America	June 2005

15. Extent and Nature of Circulation		Average No. Copies Each Issue During Preceding 12 Months	No. Copies of Single Issue Published Nearest to Filing Date
a. Total Number of Copies (Net press run)		4025	4000
b. Paid and/or Requested Circulation	(1) Paid/Requested Outside-County Mail Subscriptions Stated on Form 3541. (Include advertiser's proof and exchange copies)	2731	2598
	(2) Paid In-County Subscriptions Stated on Form 3541 (Include advertiser's proof and exchange copies)		
	(3) Sales Through Dealers and Carriers, Street Vendors, Counter Sales, and Other Non-USPS Paid Distribution	606	620
	(4) Other Classes Mailed Through the USPS		
c. Total Paid and/or Requested Circulation [Sum of 15b. (1), (2), (3), and (4)] ▲		3337	3218
d. Free Distribution by Mail (Samples, compliment-ary, and other free)	(1) Outside-County as Stated on Form 3541	72	82
	(2) In-County as Stated on Form 3541		
	(3) Other Classes Mailed Through the USPS		
e. Free Distribution Outside the Mail (Carriers or other means)			
f. Total Free Distribution (Sum of 15d. and 15e.) ▲		72	82
g. Total Distribution (Sum of 15c. and 15f.) ▲		3409	3300
h. Copies not Distributed		616	700
i. Total (Sum of 15g. and h.) ▲		4025	4000
j. Percent Paid and/or Requested Circulation (15c. divided by 15g. times 100)		98%	98%

16. Publication of Statement of Ownership
☐ Publication required. Will be printed in the December 2005 issue of this publication. ☐ Publication not required

17. Signature and Title of Editor, Publisher, Business Manager, or Owner

[signature]
John Tinucci – Executive Director of Subscription Services

Date
9/15/05

I certify that all information furnished on this form is true and complete. I understand that anyone who furnishes false or misleading information on this form or who omits material or information requested on the form may be subject to criminal sanctions (including fines and imprisonment) and/or civil sanctions (including civil penalties).

Instructions to Publishers

1. Complete and file one copy of this form with your postmaster annually on or before October 1. Keep a copy of the completed form for your records.
2. In cases where the stockholder or security holder is a trustee, include in items 10 and 11 the name of the person or corporation for whom the trustee is acting. Also include the names and addresses of individuals who are stockholders who own or hold 1 percent or more of the total amount of bonds, mortgages, or other securities of the publishing corporation. In item 11, if none, check the box. Use blank sheets if more space is required.
3. Be sure to furnish all circulation information called for in item 15. Free circulation must be shown in items 15d, e, and f.
4. Item 15h., Copies not Distributed, must include (1) newsstand copies originally stated on Form 3541, and returned to the publisher, (2) estimated returns from news agents, and (3), copies for office use, leftovers, spoiled, and all other copies not distributed.
5. If the publication had Periodicals authorization as a general or requester publication, this Statement of Ownership, Management, and Circulation must be published; it must be printed in any issue in October or, if the publication is not published during October, the first issue printed after October.
6. In item 16, indicate the date of the issue in which this Statement of Ownership will be published.
7. Item 17 must be signed.

Failure to file or publish a statement of ownership may lead to suspension of Periodicals authorization.

PS Form 3526, October 1999 (Reverse)

Changing Your Address?

Make sure your subscription changes too! When you notify us of your new address, you can help make our job easier by including an exact copy of your Clinics label number with your old address (see illustration below.) This number identifies you to our computer system and will speed the processing of your address change. Please be sure this label number accompanies your old address and your corrected address—you can send an old Clinics label with your number on it or just copy it exactly and send it to the address listed below.

We appreciate your help in our attempt to give you continuous coverage. Thank you.

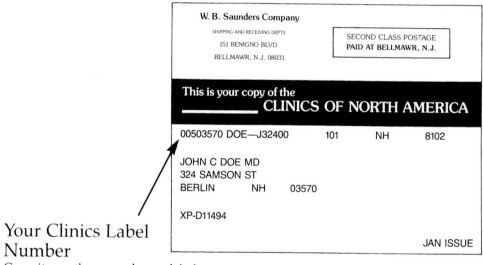

W. B. Saunders Company

SHIPPING AND RECEIVING DEPTS.

151 BENIGNO BLVD.

BELLMAWR, N.J. 08031

SECOND CLASS POSTAGE
PAID AT BELLMAWR, N.J.

This is your copy of the

_____ CLINICS OF NORTH AMERICA

00503570 DOE—J32400   101   NH   8102

JOHN C DOE MD
324 SAMSON ST
BERLIN   NH   03570

XP-D11494

JAN ISSUE

Your Clinics Label Number

Copy it exactly or send your label
along with your address to:
W.B. Saunders Company, Customer Service
Orlando, FL 32887-4800
Call Toll Free 1-800-654-2452

Please allow four to six weeks for delivery of new subscriptions and for processing address changes.